Register Now for Online Access to Your Book!

SPRINGER PUBLISHING
CONNECT™

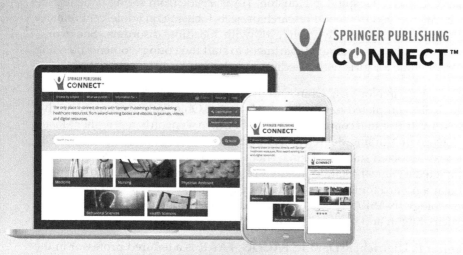

Your print purchase of *NASPAG's Protocols for Pediatric and Adolescent Gynecology: A Ready-Reference Guide for Nurses* **includes online access to the contents of your book**—increasing accessibility, portability, and searchability!

Access today at:
http://connect.springerpub.com/content/book/978-0-8261-5195-7
or scan the QR code at the right with your smartphone
and enter the access code below.

BKL4DNK3

Scan here for quick access.

If you are experiencing problems accessing the digital component of this product, please contact our customer service department at cs@springerpub.com

The online access with your print purchase is available at the publisher's discretion and may be removed at any time without notice.

Publisher's Note: New and used products purchased from third-party sellers are not guaranteed for quality, authenticity, or access to any included digital components.

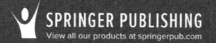

SPRINGER PUBLISHING
View all our products at springerpub.com

Jane Geyer, RN, MSN, WHNP-BC, is a board-certified nurse practitioner in women's health. She is a faculty member at the instructor level in the OB/GYN department at Baylor College of Medicine. She currently works as a nurse practitioner in the Pediatric and Adolescent Gynecology Department at Texas Children's Hospital in Houston, Texas. Aside from seeing patients, she has been involved in several research projects focusing on adolescent females with lupus and young women/girls with bleeding disorders. She works closely with the hematology department to staff the young women's bleeding disorder clinic for girls with bleeding and clotting disorders.

Jane grew up in Norwich, Ohio, and lived in the Buckeye State until graduate school. She completed her bachelor's degree at Ohio State University, with a focus in nutrition and community health. She then went on to receive her Master of Science in Nursing degree at Vanderbilt University. While at Vanderbilt, she was inducted into the Sigma Theta Tau Honor Society of Nursing. She completed a clinical rotation in adolescent gynecology and earned the Young Scholar's Award for the North American Society for Pediatric and Adolescent Gynecology (NASPAG). She has continued her involvement in NASPAG by participating in and leading the nursing SIG.

Jennifer E. Dietrich, MD, MSc, FACOG, FAAP, is a tenured professor in the Department of OB/GYN and Department of Pediatrics at Baylor College of Medicine. She is the fellowship director and division director for pediatric and adolescent gynecology. She is chief of pediatric and adolescent gynecology at Texas Children's Hospital, and became medical staff president-elect of Texas Children's Hospital in May 2019.

She grew up in Pocatello, Idaho, but education and employment led her out of the Rocky Mountains. She completed her undergraduate training with a Bachelor of Science degree in Biology at Pacific Lutheran University. She obtained her medical degree from the Medical College of Wisconsin. She completed residency in OB/GYN at Baylor College of Medicine and went on to complete her fellowship in pediatric and adolescent gynecology at the University of Louisville. She was recruited back to Baylor College of Medicine in 2007, working to build the pediatric and adolescent gynecology program.

She has been a member of the North American Society for Pediatric and Adolescent Gynecology (NASPAG) for nearly two decades and has been involved in many leadership roles within the Education Committee, NASPAG Board, ABOG Focused Practice Committee, Fellowship Directors SIG, and Ad Hoc Coding Committee; she was a past Annual Clinical and Scientific Program Meeting chair and a past president, completing her term in 2018. Finally, she currently serves as the associate editor of gynecology for the *Journal of Pediatric and Adolescent Gynecology*.

NASPAG'S PROTOCOLS FOR PEDIATRIC AND ADOLESCENT GYNECOLOGY

A READY-REFERENCE GUIDE FOR NURSES

Jane Geyer, RN, MSN, WHNP-BC

Jennifer E. Dietrich, MD, MSc, FACOG, FAAP

Editors

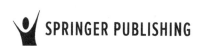

Springer Publishing Company, LLC
11 West 42nd Street, New York, NY 10036
www.springerpub.com
connect.springerpub.com/

Acquisitions Editor: Elizabeth Nieginski
Compositor: diacriTech

ISBN: 978-0-8261-5194-0
ebook ISBN: 978-0-8261-5195-7
DOI: 10.1891/9780826151957

20 21 22 23 24 / 5 4 3 2 1

The author and the publisher of this Work have made every effort to use sources believed to be reliable to provide information that is accurate and compatible with the standards generally accepted at the time of publication. Because medical science is continually advancing, our knowledge base continues to expand. Therefore, as new information becomes available, changes in procedures become necessary. We recommend that the reader always consult current research and specific institutional policies before performing any clinical procedure or delivering any medication. The author and publisher shall not be liable for any special, consequential, or exemplary damages resulting, in whole or in part, from the readers' use of, or reliance on, the information contained in this book. The publisher has no responsibility for the persistence or accuracy of URLs for external or third-party Internet websites referred to in this publication and does not guarantee that any content on such websites is, or will remain, accurate or appropriate.

Library of Congress Control Number: 2020910278

Contact us to receive discount rates on bulk purchases. We can also customize our books to meet your needs.

For more information please contact: sales@springerpub.com

Publisher's Note: **New and used products purchased from third-party sellers are not guaranteed for quality, authenticity, or access to any included digital components.**

Printed in the United States of America.

CONTENTS

CONTRIBUTORS

Kara Bendle, MSN, RN, CPN, CNL Cincinnati Children's Hospital Medical Center, Cincinnati, Ohio

Jennifer Bercaw-Pratt, MD Baylor College of Medicine, Houston, Texas

Krista Childress, MD Emory University School of Medicine and Children's Healthcare of Atlanta, Atlanta, Georgia

Jane Geyer, MSN, WHNP-BC Baylor College of Medicine, Houston, Texas

Jessica Ginn, RN, MSN, CPNP Pediatric Nurse Practitioner, Houston, Texas

Jeanette Higgins, RN, MSN, CPNP Children's Mercy Hospital, Kansas City, Missouri

Jennifer Kurkowski, MSN, WHNP-BC Baylor College of Medicine, Houston, Texas

Dana Lenobel, RN, MSN, FNP-C Nationwide Children's Hospital, Columbus, Ohio

Deborah Morse, MSN, RN, CPN, CNL Retired, Cincinnati, Ohio

Abigail Smith, PA-C, MPH Children's Healthcare of Atlanta, Atlanta, Georgia

PREFACE

This pediatric and adolescent gynecology (PAG) nurse triage book is the first of its kind because it will serve as a guide to assist nurses in efficiently addressing common patient concerns in this population. Nurses serve as the first line of communication with patients and families via telephone and computerized messages and are required to triage a wide variety of gynecologic medical questions and concerns. This triage guide has been thoughtfully constructed to approach problems from the nursing perspective. The book follows a targeted format that allows nurses to easily find and scan information on common concerns faced in this patient population.

The conditions and treatment plans in this younger population differ from adult gynecologic patients, which highlights the importance of a specialized triage guide. This guidebook differs from all other nursing resources currently available: it is the first text to focus on the specialized field of PAG.

The book addresses a multitude of common PAG patient questions and chief complaints, including acute and chronic symptoms and commonly prescribed medication side effects and use instructions. This triage book is not intended to guide advanced providers or replace physician decision-making, and it does not highlight advanced-level standards of care as outlined for practitioners. This book addresses decision-making for nurses as they approach triage concerns in this specialized patient population.

Jane Geyer, RN, MSN, WHNP-BC
Jennifer E. Dietrich, MD, MSc, FACOG, FAAP

ACKNOWLEDGMENTS

Thank you to Eduardo Lara-Torre, MD, FACOG, and the North American Society of Pediatric and Adolescent Gynecology (NASPAG) Board of Directors for their contributions and support.

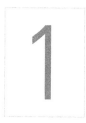

AMENORRHEA
Kara Bendle and Deborah Morse

INTRODUCTION

Amenorrhea can be defined as the absence of or abnormal cessation of periods.[1,2]

When triaging and assessing patients with complaints of amenorrhea, it is important to distinguish normal patterns of pubertal development from perceived abnormalities.[3] These common patterns can be influenced by varying fluent factors such as ethnicity, race, and socioeconomic status.[3,4] The median age of breast bud development, or thelarche, is reported to be 9.40 years.[5] Menarche, the start of menstrual periods, typically follows in approximately 2 to 3 years,[3,6,7] putting the United States median age of menarche at 12.43 years.[4]

Amenorrhea can be divided into two categories: primary amenorrhea and secondary amenorrhea.

Primary amenorrhea is defined as the complete absence of a menstrual period in a female patient if

- She is greater than 15 years of age WITH normal secondary sexual characteristics (breast development, pubertal growth spurt, pubic hair, axillary hair),[1] or
- If breast development started before the age of 10 years and it has been more than 5 years since thelarche,[1] or
- If she is 13 years of age WITHOUT secondary sexual characteristics.[1]

Primary amenorrhea can result from chromosomal abnormalities, as in Turner syndrome or androgen insensitivity syndrome (AIS), or anatomic anomalies, as in Mayer–Rokitansky–Kuster–Hauser syndrome (MRKH), imperforate hymen, or transverse vaginal septum.[1,7–9]

Secondary amenorrhea in a female patient is:

- Amenorrhea for 3 months in a patient who previously had regular periods,[1,8] or
- Amenorrhea of 6 months in patients with oligomenorrhea.[1,8]

Common causes of secondary amenorrhea include pregnancy, polycystic ovary syndrome (PCOS), hyperprolactinemia, hypothalamic disorders resulting from excess exercise, weight loss or stress, primary ovarian insufficiency (POI), thyroid disease, and chronic illness.[1,7–10]

The treatment of amenorrhea depends on the underlying cause, which is determined by patient history, physical exam, laboratory tests, and/or imaging.[1,8,9] Recommended interventions may include keeping a menstrual calendar, healthy lifestyle changes, medications, counseling, or referral to a surgical specialist.[1,7–9]

COMMON PATIENT CONCERNS

- Anxiety
- Pain

◉ KEY QUESTIONS TO ASK[1,3,7–9,11,12]

Primary Amenorrhea:

- Has the patient ever noticed any vaginal bleeding or spotting?
- Does the patient have pain? If so, is the pain constant or cyclic?
- When did the patient first note breast development?
- Is the patient sexually active? If so, is there any chance of pregnancy?
- What medications is the patient currently taking?
- Does the patient have a history of receiving chemotherapy or radiation?
- Has the patient been diagnosed with another medical condition such as kidney disease, malignancy, or a gastrointestinal disorder?
- Is there a family history of delayed puberty or late menarche?
- Does the patient notice breast discharge?
- Has the patient noticed any hair or skin changes, such as extra facial hair or acne?
- Has the patient experienced weight changes?
- Has the patient had recent changes in diet such as a weight loss plan, or new dietary restrictions?
- Has the patient's level of exercise recently increased in duration or intensity?
- Has the patient experienced any new or unusual stress?
- Does the patient experience frequent headaches or visual changes or defects
- Does the patient experience increased thirst or excessive urination?
- Does the patient have anosmia, a decreased or absent sense of smell?

Secondary Amenorrhea:

- When was the patient's first menstrual period?
- When was the patient's last menstrual period (LMP)?

- Is the patient sexually active? If so, is there any chance of pregnancy?
- What medications is the patient taking?
- Has the patient recently had a baby? If so, is the patient breastfeeding?
- Does the patient notice breast discharge?
- Has the patient noticed any hair or skin changes, such as extra facial hair or acne?
- Has the patient experienced weight changes?
- Has the patient had recent changes in diet such as a weight loss plan, or new dietary restrictions? Has the patient's level of exercise recently increased in duration or intensity?
- Has the patient experienced any new or unusual stress?

PATIENT ASSESSMENT

TABLE 1.1 Acute Symptoms of Amenorrhea

Acute Symptoms	Intervention/Delegation	Commonly Prescribed Medicine
Anxiety	Refer patient/parents to credible resources for review prior to evaluation. Provide reassurance that not all causes of amenorrhea negatively impact reproductive potential. Once the cause of amenorrhea is identified and treated, referral to a reproductive specialist is an option, if appropriate.	
Pain	Schedule urgent office visit or arrange for evaluation in the ED depending on severity and office practice guidelines. If the patient is sexually active, recommend an at-home UPT.	NSAIDs Acetaminophen Heating pads

NSAIDs, nonsteroidal anti-inflammatory drugs; UPT, urine pregnancy test.

TABLE 1.2 Chronic Symptoms of Amenorrhea

Chronic Symptoms	Intervention/Delegation	Commonly Prescribed Medicine
Pain	Schedule next available or routine office visit depending on severity of pain and office practice guidelines. Inquire on any changes in the patient's pain such as a worsening, improvement, and/or change in frequency that the pain occurs. Ask provider if updated imaging prior to an appointment is appropriate	NSAIDs Acetaminophen Heating pads

NSAIDs, nonsteroidal anti-inflammatory drugs.

➡️ **RED FLAGS**

Acute pain: This may be an indication of ectopic pregnancy, miscarriage, or menstrual obstruction.[8] Patients experiencing severe pain associated with amenorrhea or chance of pregnancy should always be referred to the ED for assessment.

Persistent pain: Pain uncontrolled by common medical therapies such as nonsteroidal anti-inflammatory drugs (NSAIDs), heat, distraction, and so on. This may also be an indication of ectopic pregnancy, miscarriage, or menstrual obstruction.[8] Patients experiencing persistently severe pain associated with amenorrhea or chance of pregnancy should always be referred to the ED for assessment.

Cyclic pain: Cyclic pain occurring monthly at approximately the same time each month, lasting approximately 1 week each episode, may be an indication of an outflow tract obstruction. If the patient is not currently in pain and is stable, then the nurse should consult with a provider to arrange an office visit and potential imaging prior to the visit. If the patient is currently in pain that is severe and/or not responding to over-the-counter medications, then the patient should be referred to the ED for assessment.

Ⓞ SPECIAL POPULATION CONSIDERATIONS

- **Cancer patients:** Schedule fertility preservation counseling **as soon as possible before** chemotherapy or radiation is initiated.[13]
- **Cancer survivors:** Predicting the extent of reproductive impairment and the window of fertility for family planning has proven challenging.[13] There is limited data on how to best use ovarian reserve markers such as anti-Mullerian hormone (AMH) in counseling young cancer survivors.[13]

COMMONLY PRESCRIBED MEDICINES

It is important to note that the approach to the evaluation and medical management of an individual with primary or secondary amenorrhea is to first determine the underlying cause for the amenorrhea, then determine the appropriate medical and pharmacologic management.[7,14] Please refer to the suggested chapters for more information.

- Birth control (Chapters 2 through 7)
- Bleeding concerns (Chapter 8)
- Breast concerns (Chapter 9)
- Dysmenorrhea (Chapter 10)
- Mayer–Rokitansky–Küster–Hauser syndrome (MRKH) (Chapter 11)
- Pelvic pain (Chapters 13 and 14)
- Polycystic ovary syndrome (Chapter 15)

▓ Positive pregnancy test (Chapter 16)
▓ Primary ovarian insufficiency (Chapter 18)

SUMMARY

▓ **If pain is currently present**, schedule urgent office visit or arrange for evaluation in ED depending on severity and office practice.

▓ **If pain has been cyclic but not currently present**, schedule next available office visit. Ask provider if imaging needs to be obtained prior to visit.

▓ **If secondary amenorrhea**, recommend home pregnancy test and **if positive** and patient is **without pain,** schedule next available office visit with provider or refer/arrange for follow up with obstetrician per office practice guidelines.

▓ If symptoms meet criteria for primary or secondary amenorrhea and **pregnancy has been ruled out,** and the patient has **no complaints of pain**, schedule routine office visit. Ask provider if testing needs to be obtained prior to visit.

▓ If symptoms **do not meet criteria for amenorrhea**, recommend documentation of symptoms (breast tenderness, mood changes, pain/cramping, bleeding) and schedule routine office visit.

RELATED PROTOCOLS

▓ Birth control (Chapters 2 through 7)
▓ Bleeding concerns (Chapter 8)
▓ Breast concerns (Chapter 9)
▓ Dysmenorrhea (Chapter 10)
▓ MRKH (Chapter 11)
▓ Pelvic pain (Chapters 13 and 14)
▓ Polycystic ovary syndrome (Chapter 15)
▓ Positive pregnancy test (Chapter 16)
▓ Primary ovarian insufficiency (Chapter 18)

References

1. Practice Committee of the American Society for Reproductive Medicine. Current evaluation of amenorrhea. *Fertil Steril.* 2008;90(suppl 5):S219–S225. doi:10.1016/j.fertnstert.2008.08.038
2. Mosby's Pocket Dictionary of Medicine. *Nursing & Health Professions.* 6th ed. St. Louis, MO: Elsevier, 2010:62
3. American College of Obstetricians and Gynecologists. ACOG committee opinion no. 651: menstruation in girls and adolescents: using the menstrual cycle as a vital sign. *Obstet Gynecol.* 2015;126:e143-146. doi:10.1097/AOG.0000000000001215
4. Chumlea WC, Schubert CM, Roche AF, et al. Age at menarche and racial comparisons in US girls. *Pediatrics.* 2003;111(1):110–103. doi:10.1542/peds.111.1.110

5. Biro FM, Greenspan LC, Galvez MP, et al. Onset of breast development in a longitudinal cohort. *Pediatrics*. 2013;132(6):1019–1027. doi:10.1542/peds.2012-3773

6. Biro FM, Huang B, Crawford PB, et al. Pubertal correlates in black and white girls. *J Pediatr*. 2006;148:234–240. doi:10.1016/j.jpeds.2005.10.020

7. North American Society for Pediatric and Adolescent Gynecology. NASPAG patient handout: amenorrhea. 2019. https://www.naspag.org/page/patienttools. Accessed February 13, 2018.

8. Klein DA, Poth MA. Amenorrhea: an approach to diagnosis and management. *Am Fam Physician*. 2013;87(11):781–788.

9. Master-Hunter T, Heiman DL. Amenorrhea: evaluation and treatment. *Am Fam Physician*. 2006;73(8):1374–1382.

10. Serri O, Chik CL, Ur E, Ezzat S. Diagnosis and management of hyperprolactinemia. *CMAJ*. 2003;169(6):575–581.

11. Gordon CM, Ackerman KE, Berga SL, et al. Functional hypothalamic amenorrhea: an endocrine society clinical practice guideline. *J Clin Endocrinol Metab*. 2017; 102(5):1413-1439. doi:10.1210/jc.2017-00131

12. Jones RE, Brashers VL, Huether SE. Alterations of hormonal regulation. In: McCance KL, Huether SE, Brashers VL, Rote NS, eds. *Pathophysiology: The Biologic Basis for Disease in Adults and Children*. 6th ed. Maryland Heights, MO: Mosby Elsevier, 2010:727–780.

13. Appiah LA, Davies MC. Late effects of childhood cancer in pediatric and adolescent gynecology practice. In: Creighton SM, Belen A, Breech L, Liao LM, eds. *Pediatric and Adolescent Gynecology: A Problem-Based Approach*. New York, NY: Cambridge University Press, 2018:132–138.

14. Crouch NS, Allen L. Primary amenorrhea in pediatric and adolescent gynecology practice: clinical evaluation. In: Creighton SM, Balen A, Breech L, Liao LM, eds. *Pediatric and Adolescent Gynecology: A Problem-Based Approach*. New York, NY.: Cambridge University Press, 2018;83–85.

2

BIRTH CONTROL: PILLS

Jane Geyer

INTRODUCTION

Combined oral contraceptives (COCs) contain two hormones, estrogen and progestin. The combined options come in the form of a pill, vaginal ring, or transdermal skin patch. These options are approximately 91% effective as contraception with typical use.[1] The combined pills are typically used for 21 to 24 days at a time, with a hormone-free interval of 4 to 7 days. Extended cycling regimens are also available to patients when desired, in which the patient has a hormone-free interval every 2 to 3 months. This will vary depending on the patient and the COC formulation the patient is using. The combined hormonal effects prevent pregnancy by inhibiting ovulation, thickening cervical mucus, and thinning the endometrial lining.

Noncontraceptive benefits:

- Menstrual regulation
- Improvement in menstrual cramps
- Lighter menstrual bleeding
- Improvement in acne/hirsutism
- Decreases risk of some cancers, including uterine and ovarian cancers
- Improvement in premenstrual syndrome (PMS)
- Prevention of ovarian cysts
- Prevention of ectopic pregnancy

The **progestin-only birth control pills (POPs),** sometimes known as the "mini-pill," contain only one progestin hormone called norethindrone. This pill works differently than the combined birth control pill, as ovulation is suppressed in approximately 50% of users.[2] This pill inhibits pregnancy by thickening cervical mucus, suppressing luteinizing hormone (LH) and follicle-stimulating hormone (FSH) peaks, thinning the endometrial lining of the uterus, and slowing the movement of the ovum through the fallopian tubes.

Noncontraceptive benefits:

- Decreases the risk of uterine cancer[3]
- May improve menstrual cramps, but has not been studied
- May lighten menstrual bleeding, but has not been studied

CLINICAL PEARL BOX

There are many different brands and types of pills on the market. It may be difficult to memorize and/or recognize every name of every pill. The COCs may contain the hormone "ethinyl estradiol" + one additional hormone. There is another type of combination pill available, which contains estradiol valerate and a progesterone. The POP types will always contain 0.35 mg of norethindrone.

COC, combined oral contraceptive; POP, progestin-only birth control pills

---

INITIATION

Birth control pills can be initiated at any time when pregnancy can reasonably be excluded. If the birth control is initiated within 5 days of onset of last menstrual period (LMP), a backup contraceptive option is not needed. When initiating pills more than 5 days after the LMP, the patient should be advised to use barrier contraception for 7 days.[1]

ADMINISTRATION

Take one tab by mouth daily at the **same time** each day.

HORMONE INTERVALS

- 21-day pill packs: Take a hormonal or "active" pill for 21 days and stop pills for 7 days. The patient should start a new pack immediately after the hormone-free interval.
- 28-day pill packs: Take active pills for 21 or 24 days (depending on pill brand) and stop pills or take inactive pills for 4 to 7 days. The patient should start a new pack immediately after the hormone-free interval.
- Extended cycling regimen with 21- to 28-day pill packs: Take an active pill daily for 3 months. Stop pills or take hormone-free pills for 7 days every 3 months. The patient should start a new pack immediately after the hormone-free interval.
- Extended cycling regimen with 91-day pill pack: Take pills daily. The final week of pills may contain a hormone, but the patient typically should expect menses during the last row of pills. The patient should start a new pack as soon as the pill pack is finished.
- The progestin-only pill comes in a pack with 28 days of active hormones and does not contain a "hormone-free" pill. The patient should take one tablet daily, and start a new pack as soon as the pill pack is finished.

TIPS FOR PROMOTING ADHERENCE

▪ Encourage the patient to set a recurring reminder or timer on the patient's phone.
▪ Encourage the patient to place the pill pack or a reminder card near her toothbrush or something that she does daily at the same time.
▪ If the patient is missing pills frequently, assist the patient in making an office visit to discuss a different contraceptive option.

COMMON PATIENT CONCERNS

▪ Missed or late doses
▪ Breakthrough or unscheduled vaginal bleeding is the most common side effect
▪ Other side effects such as breast tenderness, nausea, headaches, bloating
▪ Medication interactions

(O) KEY QUESTIONS TO ASK

Missed or late doses:
▪ How many pills were missed?
▪ Has the patient had any breakthrough bleeding?
▪ Has the patient had unprotected sex within 1 week of the missed pills?

Breakthrough or unscheduled bleeding:
▪ When did the bleeding start?
▪ How many pads or tampons has the patient been changing? How saturated are the pads or tampons?
▪ When were the pills started?
▪ Has the patient missed any doses or taken any pills late?
▪ Has the patient been sexually active? If so, has the patient missed any pills and/or has she been having unprotected intercourse?

Amenorrhea:
▪ When was the patient's LMP?
▪ Which pill formulation is the patient using?
▪ Is the patient using a cyclic or continuous pill regimen?
▪ Has the patient been sexually active? If so, has the patient missed any pills and/or has she been having unprotected intercourse?

Headaches:
▪ When did the headaches begin?
▪ Does the patient already have a history of headaches or migraines? If so, any worsening or increased frequency?

▨ Are there any other symptoms associated with the headache, including symptoms of visual disturbances during or prior to the headache?
▨ Which medications or interventions has the patient tried?

Mood changes:

▨ When did the patient first notice mood changes?
▨ When did the patient first start the contraceptive pills?
▨ Have there been any changes at home or at school that could be contributing factors?
▨ Any thoughts of harming self or others, or suicidal ideations?

Weight gain:

▨ When did the patient first notice weight gain?
▨ How much weight has the patient gained?
▨ When did the patient first start the contraceptive pills?
▨ Have there been any changes in dietary or exercise habits?
▨ Has the patient started any new medications?
▨ Are there any associated symptoms such as hair or skin changes?

COMBINED ORAL CONTRACEPTIVE PILLS

TABLE 2.1 Side Effects and Patient Concerns for Combined Oral Contraceptive Pills

Side Effects/Patient Concerns	Counseling/Intervention
Missed or late doses	**For combined OCPs:** **One missed pill or 24–<48 hours late:** ▨ Take missed dose as soon as possible. ▨ Continue taking the remainder of pills as usual. ▨ No backup contraception or EC needed. **Two or more consecutive pills missed or >48 hours since last dose:** ▨ Take most recent missed dose as soon as possible. Discard the remaining missed doses. ▨ Continue taking the remaining pills at the usual time. ▨ Use backup contraception for the next 7 days. ▨ If doses were missed during the last week of "active pills," finish taking the active pills and skip hormone-free week and immediately start a new pill pack. If the patient is unable to start a new pill pack at that time, instruct the patient to use a backup method for 7 days after new pill pack is initiated.[1] ▨ See below for breakthrough bleeding management.

(continued)

TABLE 2.1 Side Effects and Patient Concerns for Combined Oral Contraceptive Pills (*continued*)

Side Effects/Patient Concerns	Counseling/Intervention
Medication interactions	Certain medications can **decrease the efficacy** of hormonal contraceptive pills. Patients using any of these medications should be advised to use a backup method of contraception. ■ **Anticonvulsants: phenytoin, carbamazepine, barbiturates, primidone, topiramate, felbamate, or oxcarbazepine.** COCs are still safe in patients using this population and reasonable but the patient should be aware. ■ **Antimicrobials: Rifampin is the only antibiotic proven to decrease serum ethinyl estradiol and progestin levels in women taking COCs.**[1] The nurse should assist the patient in making an office visit to discuss interactions and alternative contraceptive options. By contrast, **COCs can increase lamotrigine** clearance, causing a significant decrease in serum concentrations of lamotrigine. This interaction may lead to less adequate seizure control, and the medication regimen may require adjustment.[4]
Amenorrhea	■ Amenorrhea may be the desired effect in patients using continuous or extended cycling regimens. ■ If the patient has missed any pills and patient is sexually active, recommend an at-home urine pregnancy test.
BTB or unscheduled bleeding	When using COCs cyclically: ■ The most common side effect with combined oral contraception is breakthrough bleeding. This usually resolves within the first 3 months of use.[5] If patient has been using the pills >3 months and finds the breakthrough bleeding bothersome, recommend a clinic visit to discuss alternative options with a provider. ■ Chlamydia, smoking, and missed or late pills can increase spotting and BTB. If the patient has been sexually active and has not had recent STI testing, offer/recommend an appointment.[6] ■ Provide reassurance that this is not associated with decreased efficacy of the pills in absence of late or missed pills, so encourage patients to continue with the pills.[7]

(*continued*)

TABLE 2.1 Side Effects and Patient Concerns for Combined Oral Contraceptive Pills (*continued*)

Side Effects/Patient Concerns	Counseling/Intervention
	When taking COCs pills continuously:
	▪ This is most common during first 3–6 months of use when taking pills continuously.
	▪ As long as the patient has been taking OCPs for 21 days, recommend stopping the pills for 3–4 days and restarting with a new pill pack.[7]
	▪ If bothersome to the patient, recommend a clinic visit to discuss with the provider. Persistent BTB can sometimes be affected by the dose of pill and/or progesterone component of the pill.[8–9]
	▪ Provide reassurance that this is not associated with decreased efficacy of the pills in absence of late or missed pills, so encourage patients to continue with the pills.[7]
	For either regimen (cyclic or noncyclic use) with COCs or POPs:
	For any *heavy* or *prolonged bleeding* (>7 days), please see chapter on heavy vaginal bleeding for additional assessment questions/management.
	Chlamydia, smoking, and missed or late pills can increase spotting and breakthrough bleeding. If the patient has been sexually active and has not had recent STI testing, please offer/recommend an appointment.[7]
Headaches	▪ Studies do not support strong association of headaches with COC. In patients that reported headaches with early OCP use, symptoms usually resolve within 3 months with continuation of pills.[10]
	▪ Over-the-counter NSAIDs are first-line management for most *mild to moderate* headaches.
	▪ For severe headaches, especially if unrelieved with over-the-counter medications, patients should be instructed to go to the ED for assessment.
	▪ It is important to know that migraines *with aura* are a contraindication to using estrogen.[1]
Mood changes	▪ Studies regarding mood changes are conflicting and do not strongly associate mood changes with combined hormonal contraception.[11]
	▪ Recommend clinic evaluation to further assess and to discuss alternative options.
	▪ Patients experiencing active suicidal thoughts or thoughts of harming oneself or others should always be sent to the ED for evaluation.
	▪ National suicide hotline: 1-800-273-8255

(continued)

TABLE 2.1 Side Effects and Patient Concerns for Combined Oral Contraceptive Pills (*continued*)

Side Effects/Patient Concerns	Counseling/Intervention
Nausea	■ Some clinicians may recommend taking the OCP with food and at bedtime. If the patient has tried this and is still struggling with nausea and/or vomiting from the pills, consult with the patient's provider to see if additional intervention and/or medication changes are required.
Weight gain	■ Studies do not support weight gain associated with oral contraceptive use.[12–13] ■ The patient may need to be evaluated for other causes for weight gain. Can schedule office visit and recommend continuing with the pill if the patient is doing well otherwise.

BTB, breakthrough bleeding; COCs, combined oral contraceptives; EC, emergency contraception; NSAIDs, nonsteroidal anti-inflammatory drugs; OCPs, oral contraceptive pills; POPs, progestin-only birth control pills; STI, sexually transmitted infection.

PROGESTIN-ONLY PILL

TABLE 2.2 Side Effects and Patient Concerns for the Progestin-Only Pill

Patient Concern or Side Effect	Counseling/Intervention
Missed or late doses	**If pill is taken >3 hours late:** ■ Take most recent dose as soon as possible and continue with the remainder of pills as scheduled. ■ Use backup contraception for 48 hours.[7]
Medication interactions	■ Certain medications can decrease the efficacy of hormonal contraceptive pills. Patients using any of these medications should be advised to use a backup method of contraception. ■ The nurse should assist the patient in making an office visit to discuss alternative contraceptive options. ■ Anticonvulsants including phenytoin, carbamazepine, topiramate, and barbiturates appear to reduce the efficacy of POPs. ■ Antimicrobial medications including rifampicin and rifabutin appear to reduce the efficacy of POPs.[1] ■ Lamotrigine concentrations are not thought to be affected by POPs.[1]
Amenorrhea	■ Irregular bleeding patterns and amenorrhea can be common with any progestin-only option. ■ If there is any chance of pregnancy, the nurse should recommend the patient take a pregnancy test.

(*continued*)

TABLE 2.2 Side Effects and Patient Concerns for the Progestin-Only Pill (*continued*)

Patient Concern or Side Effect	Counseling/Intervention
Breakthrough or unscheduled bleeding	■ Breakthrough bleeding and irregular bleeding patterns can be common with any progestin-only option. Taking the POP consistently at the same time each day will help to minimize BTB.[8] ■ If the patient is experiencing BTB and does not have any known contraindications to estrogen, she may want to consider the addition of estrogen, as COCs typically have less irregular bleeding patterns.[14] Recommend a clinic visit to discuss with a provider.
Headaches	■ POPs do not increase headache frequency.[15] ■ Over-the-counter NSAIDs are first-line management for most *mild to moderate* headaches. ■ Recommend the patient make an appointment with a primary care practitioner for evaluation of the headaches. ■ For severe headaches, especially if unrelieved with over the counter medications, patients should be instructed to go to the ED for assessment.
Mood changes	■ Studies are inconclusive on mood changes from the POP.[16] ■ Recommend clinic evaluation to further assess and to discuss alternative options. ■ Patients experiencing active suicidal thoughts or thoughts of harming oneself or others should always be sent to the ED for evaluation. ■ National suicide hotline: 1-800-273-8255
Nausea	■ Nausea and vomiting with contraceptive pills has been associated with the estrogen component in the pills, and therefore should not be related to the POP.[17]
Weight gain	■ The POPs have not been shown to cause weight gain.[18] ■ The patient may need to be evaluated for other causes for weight gain. Can schedule office visit and recommend continuing with the pill if the patient is doing well otherwise.

BTB, breakthrough bleeding; NSAIDs, nonsteroidal anti-inflammatory drugs; POPs, progestin-only birth control pills.

⮕ RED FLAGS

Remember **ACHES**. If a patient experiences any signs or symptoms of venous thromboembolism (VTE) or other thrombotic events, the pills should be stopped *immediately* and the patient should be instructed to proceed to the nearest ED:

TABLE 2.3 The "ACHES" Mnemonic

A	Abdominal pain (severe), cramping, vomiting
C	Chest pain, shortness of breath, radiating left arm or shoulder pain
H	Headaches, blurred vision or vision difficulty, sudden intellectual change or difficulty with speech
E	Eye changes, partial or complete vision loss
S	Swelling, pain/tenderness, erythema in upper or lower extremity.

VTE is most common in the first few months of use and gradually decreases with continued use. Risk from oral contraceptive pills (OCPs) does not completely resolve until OCPs are discontinued.[19]

⊙ SPECIAL POPULATION CONSIDERATIONS

Combined birth control pills are generally safe for the majority of young females. In most cases, they should not be started in premenarchal patients but can be initiated once menarche is achieved. Due to a slight risk of deep vein thrombosis (DVT) and/or stroke, certain patients should not be started on combined contraceptive options.

Some of the medical conditions that represent an unacceptable health risk (contraindications) to COC use include:

- Multiple risk factors for arterial cardiovascular disease
- Uncontrolled hypertension
- History of stroke or VTE
- Known thrombogenic mutations or clotting disorders
- Known ischemic heart disease
- Complicated valvular heart disease (pulmonary hypertension, risk for atrial fibrillation, history of subacute bacterial endocarditis)
- Liver disease or liver tumors
- Migraine with aura
- Breast cancer

The **risks may outweigh the benefits** in patients with:

- History of malabsorptive bariatric procedures
- Concurrent use of certain anticonvulsants and antiretrovirals (see above for medication interactions)

The POP is usually a safe option for those patients unable to use the estrogen-containing pills. Contraindications to using the progestin-only pill include:

- Breast cancer
- Liver disease or liver tumors

The **risks may outweigh the benefits** in patients with:

- History of malabsorptive bariatric procedures
- Concurrently using certain anticonvulsants and antiretrovirals (see above for medication interactions)

AFTER DISCONTINUING THE PILLS

- Return to fertility can be immediate after discontinuing the pills; if pregnancy is not desired, the patient should be instructed to return to clinic to initiate another contraceptive option and should use barrier contraception.
- Amenorrhea or irregular menses can be common the first few months after discontinuing the pills; however, if unprotected sex has occurred, the patient should rule out pregnancy if she is experiencing amenorrhea.

SUMMARY

- OCPs most often are combined with estrogen/progesterone. Patients who are unable to take COCs due to certain medical conditions may select the POP.
- Breakthrough or unscheduled vaginal bleeding is the most common side effect of birth control pills.
- Most common side effects resolve within 3 months of use.
- The nurse should be familiar with contraindications to estrogen such as migraines with aura, hypertension, or conditions that increase the risk of VTE.
- Remember ACHES:
  - Abdominal pain (severe), cramping, vomiting
  - Chest pain, shortness of breath, radiating left arm or shoulder pain
  - Headaches, blurred vision or vision difficulty, sudden intellectual change or difficulty with speech
  - Eye changes, partial or complete vision loss
  - Swelling, pain/tenderness, erythema in upper or lower extremity.

RELATED PROTOCOLS

■ Quick start initiation: Studies have shown increased adherence and decreased pregnancy rates with the "quick start" method of OCPs (Quick Start). This protocol favors the patient starting the birth control option the same day the prescription is received instead of waiting for the next menstrual cycle. Many providers may recommend this method to teenagers and adolescents.[20]

■ Office follow up: Consult with the patient's provider regarding initial follow-up visit along with routine maintenance follow up.

References

1. Curtis K, Tepper N, Jatlaoui T, et al. U.S. medical eligibility criteria for contraceptive use, 2016. *MMWR Recomm Rep*. 2016;65(3):1. Epub July 29, 2016. doi:10.15585/mmwr.rr6503a1.

2. FDA. *Orthomicronor (norethindrone)* [pacakage insert]. Raritan, NJ; Ortho-McNeil. Revised June 2008.

3. Weiderpass E, Adami HO, Baron JA, et al. Risk of endometrial cancer following estrogen replacement with and without progestins. *J Natl Cancer Inst*. 1999;91(13):1131. doi:10.1093/jnci/91.13.1131.

4. Wegner I, Edelbroek P, Bulk S, Lindhout D. Lamotrigine kinetics within the menstrual cycle, after menopause, and with oral contraceptives. *Neurology*. 2009;73(17):1388. doi:10.1212/WNL.0b013e3181bd8295.

5. Schrager S. Abnormal uterine bleeding associated with hormonal contraception. *Am Fam Physician*. May 15, 2002;65(10):2073–2080.

6. Thorneycroft I. Cycle control with oral contraceptives: a review of the literature. *Am J Obstet Gynecol*. 1999;180(2 pt 2):280. doi:10.1016/S0002-9378(99)70719-2.

7. Curtis K, Jatlaoui T, Tepper N, et al. U.S. selected practice recommendations for contraceptive use, 2016. MMWR Recomm Rep 2016; 65 (No. RR-4): 1–66. DOI: http://dx.doi.org/10.15585/mmwr.rr6504a1 external icon.

8. Endrikat J, Müller U, Düsterberg B. A twelve-month comparative clinical investigation of two low-dose oral contraceptives containing 20 micrograms ethinylestradiol/75 micrograms gestodene and 30 micrograms ethinylestradiol/75 micrograms gestodene, with respect to efficacy, cycle control, and tolerance. *Contraception*. 1997;55(3):131. doi:10.1016/S0010-7824(97)00025-5.

9. Edelman A, Koontz S, Nichols M, Jensen J. Continuous oral contraceptives: are bleeding patterns dependent on the hormones given? *Obstet Gynecol*. 2006;107(3):657. doi:10.1097/01.AOG.0000199950.64545.16.

10. Loder E, Buse D, Golub J. Headache as a side effect of combination estrogen-progestin oral contraceptives: a systematic review. *Am J Obstet Gynecol*. 2005;193(3 pt 1):636. doi:10.1016/j.ajog.2004.12.089.

11. Schaffir J, Worly B, Gur T. Combined hormonal contraception and its effects on mood: a critical review. *Eur J Contracept Reprod Health Care*. 2016;21(5):347. Epub August 15, 2016. doi:10.1080/13625187.2016.1217327.

12. Lindh I, Ellström A, Milsom I. The long-term influence of combined oral contraceptives on body weight. *Hum Reprod*. 2011;26(7):1917. doi:10.1093/humrep/der094.

13. Gallo M, Lopez L, Grimes D, Carayon F, Schulz K, Helmerhorst F. Combination contraceptives: effects on weight. *Cochrane Database Syst Rev.* 2014;1:CD003987. doi:10.1002/14651858.CD003987.pub5.
14. Belsey E. Vaginal bleeding patterns among women using one natural and eight hormonal methods of contraception. *Contraception.* 1988;38(2):181. doi:10.1016/0010-7824(88)90038-8.
15. MacGregor E. Contraception and headache. *Headache.* February 2013;53(2): 247–276. doi:10.1111/head.12035.
16. Worly B, Gur T, Schaffir J. The relationship between progestin hormonal contraception and depression: a systematic review. *Contraception.* 2018;97(6):478. Epub February 26, 2018. doi:10.1016/j.contraception.2018.01.010.
17. Goldzieher W, Moses LE, Averkin E, Scheel C, Taber BZ. A placebo-controlled, double blind cross-over investigation of the side effects attributed to oral contraceptives. *Fertil Steril.* 1971;22:609–623. doi:10.1016/S0015-0282(16)38469-2.
18. Lopez L, Ramesh S, Chen M, et al. Progestin-only contraceptives: effects on weight. *Cochrane Database Syst Rev.* 2016;8:CD008815. doi:10.1002/14651858.CD008815. pub4.
19. Lidegaard O, Lokkegaard E, Svendsen A, Agger C. Hormonal contraception and risk of venous thromboembolism: national follow-up study. *BMJ.* 2009;339:b2890. Epub August 13, 2009. doi:10.1136/bmj.b2890.
20. Westhoff C, Heartwell S, Edwards S, et al. Initiation of oral contraceptives using a quick start compared with a conventional start: a randomized controlled trial. *Obstet Gyencol.* June 2007;109(6):1270–1276. doi:10.1097/01.AOG.0000264550.41242.f2.

3

BIRTH CONTROL: TRANSDERMAL PATCH
Jane Geyer

INTRODUCTION

The birth control patch contains two hormones, estrogen and progestin. This option is approximately 91% effective as contraception with typical use[1] and is typically used for 21 days at a time, with a hormone-free interval of 7 days. Extended cycling regimens may also be available to patients when desired, in which the patient has a hormone-free interval every 2 to 3 months. The combined hormonal effects prevent pregnancy by inhibiting ovulation, thickening cervical mucus, and thinning the endometrial lining.

Noncontraceptive benefits:

- Menstrual regulation
- Improvement in menstrual cramps
- Lighter menstrual bleeding
- Improvement in acne/hirsutism
- Decreases risk of some cancers, including uterine and ovarian cancers
- Improvement in premenstrual syndrome PMS
- Prevention of ovarian cysts
- Prevention of ectopic pregnancy

INITIATION

The birth control patch can be initiated at any time when pregnancy can reasonably be excluded. If the patch is initiated within 5 days of onset of last menstrual period (LMP), a backup contraceptive option is not needed. When initiating the patch more than 5 days after the LMP, the patient should be advised to use barrier contraception for 7 days.[1]

ADMINISTRATION

The transdermal patch is applied topically and can be placed on the buttock, abdomen, upper arm, or upper torso. The breast area should be avoided due to potential concern for high concentrations of local estrogen on breast tissue. The patient should rotate patch placement sites each week to help prevent skin irritation.

The patch should be changed every 7 days on the same day of each week for 3 consecutive weeks. The patch should then be removed for 7 days for a hormone-free interval in patients that desire cyclic use.

Hormone intervals

- Traditional use: 21 days of hormones with a 7-day hormone-free interval.
- Extended cycling: 9 to 12 weeks of hormones with a 7-day hormone-free interval.

CLINICAL PEARL BOX

Tips for Promoting Adherence:

- Encourage the patient to set a recurring reminder or timer on the patient's phone.
- Encourage the patient to pick a day of the week where she is less busy and more likely to remember to change her patch.
- If the patient is frequently changing her patch late, assist the patient in making an office visit to discuss a different contraceptive option.

COMMON PATIENT CONCERNS

- Delayed/late patch changes
- Detached patch
- Skin irritation
- Patch placement sites
- Swimming and showering with the patch
- Breakthrough or unscheduled vaginal bleeding
- Other side effects such as breast tenderness, nausea, headaches, bloating
- Medication interactions

⊙ KEY QUESTIONS TO ASK

Patch changed late and/or fell off >24 hours

- When was the most recent patch placed?
- How long has the patch been off?

- Has the patient had any breakthrough bleeding?
- Has the patient had unprotected sex within one week?

Breakthrough or unscheduled bleeding

- When did the bleeding start?
- How many pads or tampons has the patient been changing? How saturated are the pads or tampons?
- When were the patches first started?
- Has the patient changed a patch late and/or had the patch fall off?
- Has the patient been sexually active? If so, has the patient changed a patch late and/or had the patch fall off?

Amenorrhea

- When was the patient's LMP?
- Is the patient using a cyclic or continuous patch regimen?
- Has the patient been sexually active? If so, has the patient changed a patch late and/or had the patch fall off?

Headaches

- When did the headaches begin?
- Does the patient already have a history of headaches or migraines? If so, has she noticed any worsening or increased frequency since starting the patch?
- Are there any other symptoms associated with the headache, including symptoms of visual disturbances during or prior to the headache?
- Which medications or interventions has the patient tried?

Mood changes

- When did the patient first notice mood changes?
- When did the patient first start the contraceptive patch?
- Have there been any changes at home or at school that could be contributing?
- Does the patient have any thoughts of harming self or others, or suicidal ideations?

Weight gain

- When did the patient first notice weight gain?
- How much weight has the patient gained?
- When did the patient first start the contraceptive patch?
- Have there been any changes in dietary or exercise habits?
- Has the patient started any new medications?
- Are there any associated symptoms such as hair or skin changes?

TABLE 3.1 Side Effects and Patient Concerns for the Birth Control Patch

Side Effects/ Patient Concerns	Counseling/Intervention
Detached patch	**If patch has been detached <48 hours.[1]** ■ Replace the patch as soon as possible. ■ If it has been less than <24 hours and the adhesive is still intact on detached patch, the patient can apply the same patch. ■ If the patch has decreased adhesiveness or if it has been off for >24 hours, apply a new patch from the box. ■ The patient can keep the same patch change day. ■ No backup contraception or EC is needed. **If the patch has been detached >48 hours.** ■ The patient should apply a new patch as soon as possible. ■ The patient can keep the same patch change day. ■ The patient should avoid sexual activity or use a backup contraceptive option for 7 days.
Delayed/ late patch placement	**If patch is changed late, <48 hours late[1]:** ■ The patient should apply a new patch as soon as possible. ■ The patient can keep the same patch change day. ■ No backup contraception or EC is usually needed unless the patient has applied a patch late during the first week of the patch cycle. In this case, the patient should avoid sexual activity or use a backup contraceptive option for 7 days. EC may be considered if the patient has had unprotected intercourse within past 5 days. **If the patch is changed late, >48 hours late[1]:** ■ The patient should apply a new patch as soon as possible. ■ The patient can keep the same patch change day. ■ The patient should avoid sexual activity or use a backup contraceptive option for 7 days. **If a patch is changed late during the third week (last week) of the cycle[1]:** ■ The patient should skip the hormone-free week and immediately apply a new patch as soon as possible. ■ The patch change day is not altered and further action is not needed. ■ If the patient is unable to immediately start a new patch, the patient should use backup contraception for 7 days after applying a new patch.

(continued)

TABLE 3.1 Side Effects and Patient Concerns for the Birth Control Patch (*continued*)

Side Effects/ Patient Concerns	Counseling/Intervention
Skin irritation	▪ Skin irritation with the patch is rare but is reported in some users.[2] ▪ If the patient reports skin irritation with the patch that is mild, recommend removing the patch and immediately placing a new patch at a different placement site. Recommend an evaluation in clinic. ▪ If the skin irritation is severe and is associated with extreme itching, redness, or swelling, this may be an allergic reaction. The patient should remove the patch and seek medical attention.
Swimming with the patch	▪ Swimming, showering/bathing, sweating, living in hot/ humid climates, and using saunas have not been shown to affect patch adherence and therefore do not increase risk of the patch falling off.[3]
Medication interactions	Due to transdermal absorption and bypass of the first pass effect, the patch is not thought to affect the efficacy of most medications including antibiotics and anticonvulsants. Most existing data focuses mainly on OCPs, so patients may be advised to use caution by using a backup method of contraception while taking[1]: ▪ Anticonvulsants: phenytoin, carbamazepine, barbiturates, primidone, topiramate, felbamate, or oxcarbazepine. COCs are still safe in patients using this population and reasonable but the patient should be aware. ▪ Antimicrobials: Rifampin is the only antibiotic proven to decrease serum ethinyl estradiol and progestin levels in women taking COCs. ▪ Antiretrovirals and protease inhibitors, including fosamprenavir. ▪ The nurse should assist the patient in making an office visit to discuss interactions and alternative contraceptive options.
Amenorrhea	▪ Amenorrhea may be the desired effect in patients using continuous or extended cycling regimens. ▪ If the patient is sexually active and may have changed a patch late and/or a patch may have fallen off, recommend an at-home UPT.
Breakthrough bleeding or unscheduled bleeding	When using the patch cyclically: ▪ Most common side effect with combined contraceptive options. This usually resolves within the first 3 months of use.[4] If the patient has been using the patch >3 months and finds the breakthrough bleeding bothersome, recommend a clinic visit to discuss alternative options with a provider.

(*continued*)

TABLE 3.1 Side Effects and Patient Concerns for the Birth Control Patch (*continued*)

Side Effects/ Patient Concerns	Counseling/Intervention
	▓ Chlamydia, smoking, and noncompliance can increase spotting and breakthrough bleeding.[5] If the patient has been sexually active and has not had recent STI testing, please offer/recommend an appointment.
	▓ Provide reassurance that this is not associated with decreased efficacy of birth control in absence of late or detached patches, so encourage patients to continue with the patch.[5]
	When using the patch continuously:
	▓ This is most common during first 3–6 months of continuous use.
	▓ As long as the patient has been using the patch for 21 days, recommend removing the patch for 4 days and restarting with a new patch.[1]
	▓ Provide reassurance that this is not associated with decreased efficacy in absence of late or missed patch, so encourage patients to continue use.
	For any *heavy* or *prolonged bleeding* (>7 days) please see chapter on vaginal bleeding for additional assessment questions/management.
Headaches	▓ Studies do not support strong association of headaches with combined contraceptive options. In patients who reported headaches with early OCP use, symptoms usually resolve with continuation of pills.[6]
	▓ Over-the-counter NSAIDs are first-line management for most *mild to moderate* headaches.
	▓ For severe headaches, especially if unrelieved with over-the-counter medications, patients should be instructed to go to the ED for assessment.
	▓ It is important to remember migraines *with aura* are a contraindication to using estrogen.
Mood changes	▓ Studies regarding mood changes are conflicting and do not strongly associate mood changes with combined hormonal contraception.[7]
	▓ Recommend clinic evaluation to further assess and to discuss alternative options.
	▓ Patients experiencing active suicidal thoughts, or thoughts of harming oneself or others, should always be sent to the ED for evaluation.
	▓ National suicide hotline: 1-800-273-8255
Weight gain	▓ Studies do not support weight gain associated with the patch.[8]
	▓ The patient may need to be evaluated for other causes for weight gain. Can schedule office visit and recommend continuing with the patch if the patient is doing well otherwise.

COCs, combined oral contraceptives; EC, emergency contraception; NSAIDs: nonsteroidal anti-inflammatory drugs; OCPs, oral contraceptive pills; STI, sexually transmitted infection; UPT, urine pregnancy test.

➡ RED FLAGS

Remember **ACHES**. If a patient experiences any signs or symptoms of venous thromboembolism (VTE) or other thrombotic events, the pills should be discontinued *immediately* and the patient should be instructed to proceed to the nearest ED:

TABLE 3.2 The "ACHES" Mnemonic

A	Abdominal pain (severe), cramping, vomiting
C	Chest pain, shortness of breath, radiating left arm, or shoulder pain
H	Headaches, blurred vision or vision difficulty, sudden intellectual change, or difficulty with speech
E	Eye changes, partial or complete vision loss
S	Swelling, pain/tenderness, erythema in upper or lower extremity

⊙ SPECIAL POPULATION CONSIDERATIONS

Birth control patches are generally safe for the majority of young females. In most cases, they should not be started in premenarchal patients but can be initiated once menarche is achieved. Due to a slight risk of deep vein thrombosis (DVT) and/or stroke, certain patients should not be started on combined contraceptive patches. Some studies have indicated that the patch may have a slightly higher risk of VTE than oral contraceptive pills (OCPs).[9–11]

Some of the medical conditions that represent an unacceptable health risk (contraindications) to patch use include:[1]

- Multiple risk factors for arterial cardiovascular disease
- Hypertension
- History of stroke or VTE
- Known thrombogenic mutations or clotting disorders
- Known ischemic heart disease
- Complicated valvular heart disease (pulmonary hypertension, risk for atrial fibrillation, history of subacute bacterial endocarditis)
- Liver disease or liver tumors
- Migraine with aura
- Breast cancer

The **risks may outweigh the benefits** in patients who are

- Concurrently using certain anticonvulsants and antiretrovirals (see above for medication interactions)

AFTER DISCONTINUING THE PATCH

■ Return to fertility can be immediate after discontinuing the patch.[2] If pregnancy is not desired, the patient should be instructed to return to clinic to initiate another contraceptive option and should use barrier contraception.

■ Amenorrhea or irregular menses can be common the first few months after discontinuing hormonal contraception; however, if unprotected sex has occurred, the patient should rule out pregnancy if she is experiencing amenorrhea.

SUMMARY

■ The contraceptive patch is combined with estrogen/progesterone.

■ The side effect profile of the patch is similar to OCPs, and most common side effects resolve within 3 months of use.

■ The nurse should be familiar with contraindications to estrogen such as migraines with aura, hypertension, or conditions that increase the risk of VTE.

■ Remember ACHES
  ● **A**bdominal pain (severe), cramping, vomiting
  ● **C**hest pain, shortness of breath, radiating left arm, or shoulder pain
  ● **H**eadaches, blurred vision or vision difficulty, a sudden intellectual change, or difficulty with speech
  ● **E**ye changes, partial or complete vision loss
  ● **S**welling, pain/tenderness, erythema in upper or lower extremity

RELATED PROTOCOLS

■ Quick start initiation: Studies have shown increased adherence and decreased pregnancy rates with the "quick start" method of birth control (Quick Start). This protocol favors the patient starting the birth control option the same day the prescription is received instead of waiting for the next menstrual cycle. Many providers may recommend this method to teenagers and adolescents.

■ Office follow up: Consult with the patient's provider regarding initial follow-up visit along with routine maintenance follow up.

References

1. Curtis K, Tepper N, Jatlaoui T, et al. U.S. Medical eligibility criteria for contraceptive use, 2016. *MMWR Recomm Rep.* 2016;65(3):1. Epub July 29, 2016. doi:10.15585/mmwr.rr6503a1
2. Ortho Evra (Norelgestromin/Ethinyl Estradiol Transdermal System). *Product Labeling*. Titusville, NJ: Janssen Ortho, LLC; Revised May 2018.

3. Zacur H, Hedon B, Mansour D, Shangold G, Fisher A, Creasy G. Integrated summary of Ortho Evra/Evra contraceptive patch adhesion in varied climates and conditions. *Fertil Steril.* 2002;77(2 suppl 2):S32. doi:10.1016/s0015-0282(01)03262-9

4. Schrager S. Abnormal uterine bleeding associated with hormonal contraception. *Am Fam Physician.* May 15, 2002;65(10):2073-2080

5. Thorneycroft I. Cycle control with oral contraceptives: a review of the literature. *Am J Obstet Gynecol.* 1999;180(2 pt 2):280. doi:10.1016/s0002-9378(99)70719-2

6. Loder E, Buse D, Golub J. Headache as a side effect of combination estrogen-progestin oral contraceptives: a systematic review. *Am J Obstet Gynecol.* 2005;193(3 pt 1):636. doi:10.1016/j.ajog.2004.12.089

7. Schaffir J, Worly B, Gur T. Combined hormonal contraception and its effects on mood: a critical review. *Eur J Contracept Reprod Health Care.* 2016;21(5):347. Epub August 15, 2016. doi:10.1080/13625187.2016.1217327

8. Gallo MF, Lopez LM, Grimes DA, Carayon F, Schulz KF, Helmerhorst FM. Combination contraceptives: effects on weight. *Cochrane Database Syst Rev.* January 29, 2014;(1):CD003987. 58–59. doi:10.1002/14651858.CD003987.pub5

9. Johnson J, Lowell J, Badger G, Rosing J, Tchaikovski S, Cushman M. Effects of oral and transdermal hormonal contraception on vascular risk markers: a randomized controlled *trial. Obstet Gynecol.* 2008;111(2 pt 1):278. doi:10.1097/AOG.0b013e 3181626d1b

10. Kluft C, Meijer P, LaGuardia K, Fisher AC. Comparison of a transdermal contraceptive patch vs. oral contraceptives on hemostasis variables. *Contraception.* 2008;77(2):77. Epub January 11, 2008. doi:10.1016/j.contraception.2007.10.004

11. Douketis J, Ginsberg J, Holbrook A, Crowther M, Duku E, Burrows R. A reevaluation of the risk for venous thromboembolism with the use of oral contraceptives and hormone replacement therapy. *Arch Intern Med.* 1997;157(14):1522. doi:10.1001/arc hinte.1997.00440350022002

4

BIRTH CONTROL: VAGINAL RING

Dana Lenobel

INTRODUCTION

The vaginal ring is a rubber-free, silicone birth control that is colorless and nonbiodegradable. It will not dissolve in the body. This ring is easy to insert and is placed anywhere in the vagina that feels comfortable. It was Food and Drug Administration (FDA) approved in 2001.[1]

The ring releases two hormones: 120 mcg of the progestin etonogestrel and 15 mcg of ethinyl estradiol per day.[2] The hormones are slowly and constantly released into the vagina, preventing ovulation. The hormones also thicken the cervical mucus to keep sperm from reaching a fertilized egg and inhibit endometrial growth.[1] When used as directed the ring is 98% effective.[2]

The advantages of the ring include the avoidance of gastrointestinal metabolism, no daily dosing, and a rapid return to ovulation after discontinuation.[3]

INITIATION

The vaginal ring can be initiated at any time as long as pregnancy can reasonably be excluded. If the vaginal ring is initiated within 5 days of onset of last menstrual period (LMP), a backup contraceptive option is not needed. When initiating the ring more than 5 days after the LMP, the patient should be advised to use barrier contraception for 7 days or abstain from sexual intercourse.[4]

ADMINISTRATION

Cyclic ring use regimen

- Place in the vagina and leave in place for three weeks.
- On the fourth week, the ring is removed for one week and a menses occurs. Then a new ring is placed within 7 days.
- It is important to remove and reinsert the ring on the same day of the week and at the same time to avoid unwanted pregnancy.[2]

Extended use regimen

- The ring is kept in place for 4 weeks (with no hormone-free week) and then removed, and a new one is placed on the same day.
- If a ring is left in place for longer than 4 weeks, the patient may not be protected against unwanted pregnancy.[2]
- Using the ring in a continuous fashion will most likely skip the patient's menses; however, breakthrough bleeding is not uncommon.

CLINICAL PEARL BOX

If the ring is used in a continuous fashion where it is changed every 4 weeks, ovulation is still inhibited. This continuous use does not decrease the contraceptive effectiveness.[3]

Points to consider while handling and inserting/removing the ring:

- Once the ring is in the vagina there is no wrong position. The ring will not get lost into the body. If a patient feels discomfort, the ring is most likely not inserted completely into the vagina. If discomfort is felt, advise the patient to use a clean finger to push the ring as far into the vagina as possible. The position of the ring does not affect contraceptive efficacy.[5]
- The ring does not require refrigeration for storage. Store the ring at room temperature and not in direct sunlight.[2]
- Do not use more than one ring at a time.
- The ring does not need to be removed during intercourse, however, the ring can be removed up to 3 hours without interfering with contraceptive efficacy.[2]
- If the ring is taken out or falls out and it has been less than 3 hours out of the vagina, the patient should wash it under cool or warm water and place it back into the vagina.[5]
- A tampon applicator can be used to assist the patient with inserting the ring.

SIDE EFFECTS

Systemic

- It is less common to experience breast tenderness and nausea after ring initiation when compared to oral contraceptive pills (OCPs).[6,7] Breast tenderness and nausea are due to estrogen exposure.
- There are no differences in weight gain or headaches with the ring when compared to OCPs.[3,6–9]
- There are no significant changes in blood chemistries, hematologic indices, thyroid function, lipid levels, or mood changes while using the ring.[10,11]

Local

- There is no increased risk for acquiring vaginal or cervical infections with the use of vaginal rings.[12,13] In contrast to OCP users, vaginal ring users typically report increased vaginal wetness and vaginal discharge, but this does not typically require treatment or ring discontinuation.[14]
- Cycle control is equivalent or superior when using the ring compared to OCPs and transdermal patches.[3,15,16]
- Reduction in volume loss during menses while using the ring is similar to use with OCPs.[5]
- Less than 3% of users report ring expulsion, feeling the ring, or concerns during intercourse.[17]

COMMON PATIENT CONCERNS

- Delayed/late ring removals
- Breakthrough or unscheduled vaginal bleeding
- Amenorrhea
- Headaches
- Mood changes
- Weight gain
- Vaginal concerns such as irritation, discharge, and/or discomfort

(O) KEY QUESTIONS TO ASK

Missed or late doses

- When was the ring placed?
- How long has the ring been removed?
- Has the patient had any breakthrough bleeding?
- Has the patient had unprotected sex within the past week? Could she be pregnant?

Breakthrough or unscheduled bleeding

- When did the bleeding start?
- How many pads or tampons has the patient been changing? How saturated are the pads or tampons?
- When was the ring first started?
- Has the patient removed or placed a ring late?
- Has the patient been sexually active? If so, has the patient removed or placed a ring recently?

Amenorrhea

- When was the patient's LMP?
- Is the patient using a cyclic or continuous ring regimen?
- Has the patient been sexually active? If so, has the patient removed or placed a ring lately?

Headaches

- When did the headaches begin?
- Does the patient already have a history of headaches or migraines? If so, any worsening or increased frequency?
- Any other symptoms associated with the headache, including visual changes prior to onset of the headaches?
- Which medications or interventions has the patient tried?

Mood changes

- When did the patient first notice mood changes?
- When did the patient first start the vaginal ring?
- Have there been any changes at home or at school that could be contributing factors?
- Any thoughts of harming self or others? Any suicidal ideation?

Weight gain

- When did the patient first notice weight gain?
- How much weight has the patient gained?
- When did the patient first start the vaginal ring?
- Have there been any changes in dietary or exercise habits?
- Has the patient started any new medications?
- Are there any associated symptoms such as hair or skin changes?

TABLE 4.1 Side Effects and Patient Concerns for the Vaginal Ring

Side Effects/ Patient Concerns	Counseling/Interventions
Delayed insertion of ring Delayed removal of ring	**<48 hours since a ring should have been reinserted:** - Insert ring as soon as possible and no additional contraceptive protection is needed. - Keep the ring in until scheduled ring removal day. - No backup contraception or EC needed but can be considered if delayed insertion occurred earlier in the cycle or in the last week of the previous cycle.

(continued)

TABLE 4.1 Side Effects and Patient Concerns for the Vaginal Ring (*continued*)

Side Effects/ Patient Concerns	Counseling/Interventions
	≥48 hours since a ring should have been inserted: ▪ Insert ring as soon as possible. ▪ Use backup contraception or avoid intercourse until a ring has been in place for seven consecutive days.
	▪ If the ring removal occurred in the third week of ring use: 　1. Omit the hormone-free week by finishing the third week of ring use and start a new ring right away. 　2. If unable to start a new ring right away, use backup method or avoid intercourse until a new ring has been in place for 7 days in a row. ▪ EC should be considered if delayed insertion occurred within the first week of ring use and unprotected intercourse occurred in the last 5 days.[4,18] ▪ If the ring has been in place more than 3 but ≤5 weeks: 　1. The ring is removed, and a new one is inserted after a 1-week ring-free interval. 　2. The patient can also immediately insert a new ring without using a 1-week ring-free interval, although she may have breakthrough bleeding.[5] ▪ If the ring has been in place for >5 weeks: 　1. The old ring is removed, a new ring is inserted, **and** back-up contraception is advised until the new ring has been in place for 7 days.[5]
Breakthrough bleeding or unscheduled bleeding	▪ Most common side effect with combined hormonal contraception. This usually resolves within the first 3 months of use. ▪ Provide reassurance that this is not associated with decreased efficacy of the ring in absence of late insertion. ▪ Unscheduled intermenstrual bleeding can also be a sign of sexually transmitted infection(s). If the patient has been sexually active and has not had recent STI testing, offer/recommend an appointment. ▪ For heavy or prolonged bleeding (>7 days), please see chapter on heavy vaginal bleeding for additional information.
Amenorrhea	▪ May be desired effect in those patients using continuous or extended cycling regimens. ▪ If late insertion or removal (see above) and patient is sexually active, recommend an at-home urine pregnancy test.
Headaches	▪ Studies do not support strong association of headaches with combined hormonal contraception. ▪ Over-the-counter NSAIDs are first-line management for most *mild to moderate* headaches.

(*continued*)

TABLE 4.1 Side Effects and Patient Concerns for the Vaginal Ring (*continued*)

Side Effects/ Patient Concerns	Counseling/Interventions
	■ For severe headaches, especially if unrelieved with over the counter medications, patients should be seen immediately by their primary care provider. If unable to do so, patients should be instructed to go to the ED for assessment.
	■ It is important to remember migraines with aura are a contraindication to using estrogen.[18]
	■ See red flag box below for **ACHES**
Mood changes	■ Studies regarding mood changes are conflicting and do not strongly associate mood changes with combined hormonal contraception.[19]
	■ The controlled-release delivery with the ring avoids daily fluctuations in hormones.[3]
	■ Exposure to ethinyl estradiol with the ring is approximately half of that when compared to a combination birth control pill.[3]
	■ Recommend clinical evaluation to further assess and to discuss alternative options.
	■ Patients experiencing active thoughts of harming oneself or others should always be sent to the ED for immediate evaluation.
	■ National Suicide Prevention Lifeline: 1-800-273-8255
Weight gain	■ Studies do not support weight gain associated with combined hormonal contraceptive use.[20]
	■ Patient may need to be evaluated for other causes for weight gain. Schedule office visit and recommend continuing with ring if the patient is doing well otherwise.
Vaginal concerns	■ There is only one size of the ring and a patient does not need to be fitted.
	■ A patient can have intercourse with the ring in place.
	■ Rare cases of toxic shock syndrome have been reported with the ring.[10]
	■ Tampons may be used during menses as they will not interfere with absorption of hormones from the ring when it is replaced.[5]
	■ Use of spermicides, water-based lubricants, and water-based vaginal medications for yeast and bacterial vaginosis are safe while using the ring. The oil-based miconazole suppositories can increase hormone levels.[2]
	■ The ring can interfere with other barrier methods including the cervical cap, female condom, and diaphragm.

EC, emergency contraception; STI, sexually transmitted infections.

➡ RED FLAGS

Remember **ACHES**. If a patient experiences any signs or symptoms of venous thromboembolism (VTE) or other thrombotic events, the hormonal contraceptive method should be stopped *immediately* and patient should be instructed to proceed to the nearest ED:

TABLE 4.2 The "ACHES" Mnemonic

A	Abdominal pain (severe), cramping, vomiting
C	Chest pain, shortness of breath, radiating left arm or shoulder pain
H	Headaches, blurred vision or change in vision, sudden intellectual change, or difficulty with speech
E	Eye changes, partial or complete vision loss
S	Swelling, pain/tenderness, erythema in upper or lower extremity

⊙ SPECIAL POPULATION CONSIDERATIONS

The vaginal ring is generally safe for the majority of young females. In most cases, they should not be started in premenarchal patients but can be initiated once menarche is achieved. Due to a slight risk of a VTE and/or stroke, certain patients should not be started on combined contraceptive options. **Some of the medical conditions that represent an unacceptable health risk (contraindications) to the use of the vaginal ring include the following:**

- Multiple risk factors for arterial cardiovascular disease
- Hypertension
- History of stroke or VTE
- Known thrombogenic mutations or clotting disorders
- Known ischemic heart disease
- Complicated valvular heart disease
- Liver disease or liver tumors
- Migraine with aura
- Breast cancer
- History of malabsorptive bariatric procedures
- Concurrent use of certain anticonvulsants and antiretrovirals

Obese patients: It is unknown if the efficacy of the vaginal ring is reduced with women with a BMI of ≥30.[5] From a VTE standpoint, the vaginal ring is safer than the pregnant or postpartum periods in this population.

Postpartum patients: It is best to initiate at least 21 days postpartum to reduce the risk of thromboembolic events.[4,18] Progestin-only options are typically preferred for patients while breastfeeding, as this should not interfere with milk supply.

Postabortion patients: The Centers for Disease Control and Prevention (CDC) supports initiating the ring within 7 days or the day of an abortion procedure.[2,4]

Diabetes, impaired glucose tolerance: Patients with insulin resistance or increased risk for insulin resistance are more likely to have increased insulin levels with OCP use when compared to vaginal ring users.[21]

AFTER DISCONTINUING THE VAGINAL RING

- Return to fertility can be immediate after discontinuing the vaginal ring. If pregnancy is not desired, the patient should be instructed to return to clinic to initiate another contraceptive option and should use barrier contraception.
- Amenorrhea or irregular menses can be common the first few months after discontinuing hormonal contraception; however, if unprotected intercourse has occurred, then pregnancy should be ruled out.

SUMMARY

- The contraceptive vaginal ring is a combined estrogen and progestin method.
- The nurse should be familiar with contraindications to estrogen such as migraines with aura, hypertension, or conditions that increase the risk of VTE.
- Remember ACHES
  - Abdominal pain (severe), cramping, vomiting
  - Chest pain, shortness of breath, radiating left arm or shoulder pain
  - Headaches, blurred vision or vision change, a sudden intellectual change, or difficulty with speech
  - Eye changes, partial or complete vision loss
  - Swelling, pain/tenderness, erythema in upper or lower extremity

RELATED PROTOCOLS

- Quick start initiation: Studies have shown increased adherence and decreased pregnancy rates with the "quick start" method of birth control. This protocol favors the patient starting the vaginal ring option the same day the prescription is received (even during the visit if a sample is available), instead of waiting for the next menstrual cycle. Many providers may recommend this method to teenagers and adolescents.

TRICKS FOR HELPING PATIENTS REMEMBER TO CHANGE THE VAGINAL RING ON TIME

- Encourage the patient to set a reminder on her phone.
- Encourage the patient to pick a day of the week where she is less busy and more likely to remember to change her vaginal ring.
- If the patient is frequently changing her ring late, assist the patient in making an office visit to discuss a different contraceptive option.

References

1. Gupta N, Corrado S, Goldstein M. Hormonal contraception for the adolescent. *Pediatr Rev.* 2008;29:386. doi:10.1542/pir.29-11-386
2. Nuvaring [package insert]. Whitehouse Station, NJ. Merck and Co, Inc.; 2001-2018. http://www.merck.com/product/usa/pi_circulars/n/nuvaring/nuvaring_pi.pdf. Accessed May 17, 2018.
3. Bjarnadóttir RI, Tuppurainen M, Killick SR. Comparison of cycle control with a combined contraceptive vaginal ring and oral levonorgestrel/ethinyl estradiol. *Am J Obstet Gynecol.* 2002;186:389. doi:10.1067/mob.2002.121103
4. Curtis KM, Tepper NK, Jatlaoui TC, et al. U.S. medical eligibility criteria for contraceptive use, 2016. *MMWR Recomm Rep.* 2016;65:1-104. doi:10.15585/mmwr.rr6503a1
5. Kerns J, Darney PD. *Hormonal contraceptive vaginal rings* [UpToDate]. https://www.uptodate.com/contents/hormonal-contraceptive-vaginal-rings?search=hormonal%20contraceptive&source=search_result&selectedTitle=3~150&usage_type=default&display_rank=3. Accessed May 17, 2019.
6. Ahrendt HJ, Nisand I, Bastianelli C, et al. Efficacy, acceptability and tolerability of the combined contraceptive ring, NuvaRing, compared with an oral contraceptive containing 30 microg of ethinyl estradiol and 3 mg of drospirenone. *Contraception.* 2006;74:451. doi:10.1016/j.contraception.2006.07.004
7. Sabatini R, Cagiano R. Comparison profiles of cycle control, side effects and sexual satisfaction of three hormonal contraceptives. *Contraception.* 2006;74:220. doi:10.1016/j.contraception.2006.03.022
8. Milsom I, Lete I, Bjertnaes A, et al. Effects on cycle control and bodyweight of the combined contraceptive ring, NuvaRing, versus an oral contraceptive containing 30 microg ethinyl estradiol and 3 mg drospirenone. *Hum Reprod.* 2006;21:2304. doi:10.1093/humrep/del162
9. O'Connell KJ, Osborne LM, Westhoff C. Measured and reported weight change for women using a vaginal contraceptive ring vs. a low-dose oral contraceptive. *Contraception.* 2005;72:323. doi:10.1016/j.contraception.2005.05.008
10. Nanda K. Contraceptive patch and vaginal contraceptive ring. In: Hatcher RA, Trussell, J, Nelson, AL, et al., eds. *Contraceptive Technology.* 19th ed. New York, NY: Ardent Media; 2007:271.
11. Schafer JE, Osborne LM, Davis AR, Westhoff C. Acceptability and satisfaction using quick start with the contraceptive vaginal ring versus an oral contraceptive. *Contraception.* 2006;73:488. doi:10.1016/j.contraception.2005.11.003

12. Polis CB, Phillips SJ, Curtis KM, et al. Hormonal contraceptive methods and risk of HIV acquisition in women: a systematic review of epidemiological evidence. *Contraception.* 2014;90:360. doi:10.1016/j.contraception.2014.07.009

13. De Seta F, Restaino S, De Santo D, et al. Effects of hormonal contraception on vaginal flora. *Contraception.* 2012;86:526. doi:10.1016/j.contraception.2012.02.012

14. Lopez LM, Grimes DA, Gallo MF, et al. Skin patch and vaginal ring versus combined oral contraceptives for contraception. *Cochrane Database Syst Rev.* 2013;CD003552. doi:10.1002/14651858.CD003552.pub4

15. Vercellini P, Barbara G, Somigliana E, et al. Comparison of contraceptive ring and patch for the treatment of symptomatic endometriosis. *Fertil Steril.* 2010;93:2150. doi:10.1016/j.fertnstert.2009.01.071

16. Westhoff C, Osborne LM, Schafer JE, Morroni C. Bleeding patterns after immediate initiation of an oral compared with a vaginal hormonal contraceptive. *Obstet Gynecol.* 2005;106:89. doi:10.1097/01.AOG.0000164483.13326.59

17. Roumen FJ, Apter D, Mulders TM, Dieben TO. Efficacy, tolerability and acceptability of a novel contraceptive vaginal ring releasing etonogestrel and ethinyl oestradiol. *Hum Reprod.* 2001;16:469. doi:10.1093/humrep/16.3.469

18. Curtis KM, Jatlaoui TC, Tepper NK, et al. U.S. Selected practice recommendations for contraceptive use, 2016. *MMWR Recomm Rep.* 2016;65:1-66. doi:10.15585/mmwr.rr6504a1

19. Schaffir J, Worly B, Gur T. Combined hormonal contraception and its effects on mood: a critical review. *Eur J Contracept Reprod Health Care.* 2016;21(5):347. Epub August 2016. doi:10.1080/13625187.2016.1217327

20. Lindh I, Ellström A, Milsom I. The long-term influence of combined oral contraceptives on body weight. *Hum Reprod.* 2011;26(7):1917. doi:10.1093/humrep/der094

21. Cagnacci A, Ferrari S, Tirelli A, et al. Route of administration of contraceptives containing desogestrel/etonorgestrel and insulin sensitivity: a prospective randomized study. *Contraception.* 2009;80:34. doi:10.1016/j.contraception.2009.01.012

5

BIRTH CONTROL: INJECTION
Jennifer Kurkowski

INTRODUCTION

Depot medroxyprogesterone acetate (DMPA) is an injectable, progestin-only contraceptive that provides effective, reversible contraception. It comes in two doses (DMPA, 150 mg intramuscularly or 104 mg subcutaneously). The only difference between these two formulations is the route of administration. It is highly effective, with only six out of 100 women becoming pregnant in the first year of use with typical use.[1]

Noncontraceptive benefits include but are not limited to

- Improvement in menstrual cramps
- Lighter menstrual bleeding
- Improvement in menstrual-related hygiene and/or menstrual suppression in patients with special needs[2]
- Reduction of sickle cell crises[3]
- Potential reduction of menstrual-related seizures[4]
- Prevention of endometrial hyperplasia
- Prevention of some types of ovarian cysts (hemorrhagic)[5]

INITIATION

DMPA can be initiated at any time when pregnancy can be reasonably excluded. If hormonal birth control is initiated within 5 days of the onset of the last menstrual period (LMP), a backup contraceptive option is not needed. When initiating DMPA more than 5 days after the LMP, the patient should be advised to use barrier contraception for 7 days.[1]

FREQUENCY OF DOSING

It is given every 11 to 13 weeks but can be given up to 15 weeks between injections.[1] Injections given after 15 weeks are considered late and additional contraceptive measures may be required.

CLINICAL PEARL BOX

Injections given after 15 weeks are considered late, and additional contraceptive measures may be required.

DISCONTINUING DMPA

The return to fertility after discontinuing DMPA may be delayed. In some patients, it may take up to 18 months to return to ovulatory cycles.[1]

COMMON PATIENT CONCERNS

- Irregular bleeding
- Amenorrhea
- Missed or late injections
- Weight gain
- Mood changes

⊙ KEY QUESTIONS TO ASK

For irregular bleeding

- When was DMPA initiated?
- When was the most recent injection received?
- When did the breakthrough bleeding start? How heavy is the bleeding?
- Has the patient had any new sexual partners or unprotected intercourse?

Late or missed injections

- When was the last dose of DMPA given?
- Is the patient sexually active? If so, has she had any unprotected intercourse?
- Has the patient experienced any breakthrough bleeding?
- When was the patient's LMP?

Mood changes

- When did the patient first notice mood changes?
- When did the patient first start the injection?
- Have there been any changes at home or at school that could be contributing factors?
- Is the patient having thoughts of harming self or others, or suicidal ideations?

Weight gain

- When did the patient first notice weight gain?
- How much weight has the patient gained?
- When did the patient first start the injection?
- Have there been any changes in dietary or exercise habits?
- Has the patient started any new medications?
- Are there any associated symptoms such as hair or skin changes?

PATIENT ASSESSMENT

TABLE 5.1 Acute Symptoms and Patient Concerns for the Birth Control Shot

Acute Symptoms/ Patient Concerns	Intervention/Delegation
Amenorrhea	- Reassure the patient that menstrual changes occur in all patients who receive DMPA.[6] Amenorrhea is a common side effect. - Amenorrhea may be the desired effect for patients using the injection for menstrual suppression or lighter menstrual bleeding.
Breakthrough bleeding/Irregular bleeding	- Reassure the patient that menstrual changes occur in all patients who receive DMPA.[6] - Reassure patient that within the first months of DMPA use, irregular bleeding is very common.[6] - The frequency and duration of the irregular bleeding will likely decrease with increasing duration of use.[6] - If the bleeding is unacceptable to the patient, they should make a clinic visit to discuss alternative options. - Some clinicians may recommend giving injections earlier than every 11 weeks in order to help minimize breakthrough bleeding. - If clinically indicated, consider STI testing.
Missed or late injections	- Depo Provera can be given 2 weeks late without any intervention (15 weeks from last injection).[1] - If the patient is more than 2 weeks late (>15 weeks from the last injection) for a repeat DMPA injection, she can still get another injection if pregnancy can be reasonably excluded. The patient should be advised to use a backup contraceptive method for the next 7 days. - Emergency contraception may need to be considered if unprotected intercourse has occurred in the past 3–5 days (see unprotected intercourse chapter).
Medication interactions	- DMPA has fewer drug interactions compared to other forms of contraception. - The Centers for Disease Control and Prevention (CDC) does not have any restriction with coadministration of other drugs.[1]

DMPA, depot medroxyprogesterone acetate; STI, sexually transmitted infection.

TABLE 5.2 Chronic Symptoms for the Birth Control Shot

Chronic Symptoms	Intervention/Delegation
Decreased bone density	▪ DMPA has been shown to decrease bone mineral density with each dose given in the first 2 years of use.[7] ▪ The nurse should review calcium and vitamin D supplementation recommendations with each patient. ▪ The nurse should encourage weight-bearing exercise to help protect bone density and to offset weight gain side effects with DMPA. ▪ The nurse should provide reassurance that advantages outweigh the risks of skeletal harm in most patients using DMPA.
Mood changes	▪ Review studies have not shown any consistent findings with DMPA and mood changes.[8] ▪ Recommend clinic evaluation to further assess and to discuss alternative options. ▪ Patients experiencing active suicidal thoughts, or thoughts of harming oneself or others, should always be sent to the ED for evaluation. ▪ National suicide hotline: 1-800-273-8255
Weight gain	▪ Weight gain is a common side effect of DMPA. ▪ A recent study showed that DMPA users who gained >5% of baseline body weight within 6 months of starting DMPA appeared to be at increased risk of weight gain over the following 2–3 years.[9] ▪ The nurse can encourage the patient to choose more nutrient-dense foods as small studies have suggested improving the quality of diet can help to prevent weight gain.[10] ▪ If weight gain is unacceptable another contraceptive method should be considered, and a clinic visit should be scheduled.

DMPA, depot medroxyprogesterone acetate.

➡ RED FLAGS

Heavy vaginal bleeding: If the patient is bleeding heavily and/or reports experiencing signs and symptoms of anemia, the patient should be referred to the ED for evaluation.

⊙ SPECIAL POPULATION CONSIDERATIONS

▪ **Overweight or obese patients**: Efficacy is not impacted by high body mass index (BMI).[11] DMPA should be used with caution in patients who are already overweight, as it can lead to increased weight gain.

▪ **Postabortion**: DMPA can be used immediately postabortion.[1]

- **Menstrual suppression:** Some special needs patients use DMPA for menstrual suppression. Rates for amenorrhea with DMPA are 50% to 75% and can increase over time.[1]
- **Immunosuppression:** Clinicians should weigh the risk versus benefits when deciding on whether to use DMPA versus an alternative contraceptive in women with risk factors for osteoporosis such as those on corticosteroids.[12]
- **Seizure Disorder:** DMPA appears to have some intrinsic anti-seizure effects. For this reason, DMPA may be a good option in those patients with seizure disorder. Enzyme-inducing anticonvulsants do not seem to affect DMPA.[1]
- **Immobile patients:** Evidence regarding skeletal health in immobilized patients using DMPA has not been well-studied. DMPA is still commonly used in these patients as it can be advantageous if menstrual suppression is needed and when estrogen-based contraceptives should not be used due to risk of thrombosis.

CONTRAINDICATIONS TO USING DMPA

According to the CDC guidelines, patients should not use DMPA who have the following conditions[1]:

- Patients who are pregnant
- Patients with breast cancer
- Patients with severe cirrhosis, hepatocellular adenoma, hypertension
- Patients with unexplained vaginal bleeding

SUMMARY

- DMPA is typically dosed every 11 to 13 weeks. It can be given up to 15 weeks between injections.[1]
- Injections given after 15 weeks are considered late, and additional contraceptive measures may be required.
- Irregular bleeding and amenorrhea are common side effects.
- Weight gain is a common side effect.

RELATED PROTOCOLS

- Quick start initiation from the CDC[1]
- Chapter 8: Abnormal Uterine Bleeding
- Chapter 20: Unprotected Intercourse

References

1. Curtis KM, Tepper NK, Jatlaoui TC, et al. U.S. Medical Eligibility Criteria for Contraceptive Use, 2016. *MMWR Recomm Rep.* 2016;65(3):1. Epub 2016 Jul 29. doi:10.15585/mmwr.rr6503a1

2. Elkins TE, Gafford LS, Wilks CS, Muram D, Golden G. A model clinic approach to the reproductive health concerns of the mentally handicapped. *Obstet Gynecol.* 1986;68(2):185.

3. Manchikanti A, Grimes DA, Lopez LM, Schulz KF. Steroid hormones for contraception in women with sickle cell disease. *Cochrane Database Syst Rev.* 2007:CD006261. doi:10.1002/14651858.CD006261.pub2

4. Mattson RH, Cramer JA, Caldwell BV, Siconolfi BC. Treatment of seizures with medroxyprogesterone acetate: preliminary report. *Neurology.* 1984;34(9):1255. doi:10.1212/WNL.34.9.1255

5. Sönmezer M, Atabekoğlu C, Cengiz B, Dökmeci F, Cengiz SD. Depot-medroxyprogesterone acetate in anticoagulated patients with previous hemorrhagic corpus luteum. *Eur J Contracept Reprod Health Care.* 2005;10(1):9. doi:10.1080/13625180400020952

6. DEPO-PROVERA- medroxyprogesterone acetate injection. http://labeling.pfizer.com/ShowLabeling.aspx?id=522 (Accessed on May 11, 2019).

7. Clark MK, Sowers MR, Nichols S, Levy B. Bone mineral density changes over two years in first-time users of depot medroxyprogesterone acetate. *Fertil Steril.* Dec, 2004;82(6):1580–1586. doi:10.1016/j.fertnstert.2004.04.064

8. Civic D, Scholes D, Ichikawa L, et al. Depressive symptoms in users and non-users of depot medroxyprogesterone acetate. *Contraception.* 2000;61(6):385. doi:10.1016/S0010-7824(00)00122-0

9. Steenland MW, Zapata LB, Brahmi D, Marchbanks PA, Curtis KM. Appropriate follow up to detect potential adverse events after initiation of select contraceptive methods: a systematic review. *Contraception.* May, 2013;87(5):611–624. Epub 2012. doi:10.1016/j.contraception.2012.09.017

10. Lange HL, Belury MA, Secic M, Thomas A, Bonny AE. Dietary intake and weight gain among adolescents on depot medroxyprogesterone acetate. *J Pediatric Adolesc Gynecol.* Jun, 2015;28(3):139-143. doi:10.1016/j.jpag.2014.04.004. Epub 2014 May 5

11. Segall-Gutierrez P, Taylor D, Liu X, Stanzcyk F, Azen S, Mishell DR Jr. Follicular development and ovulation in extremely obese women receiving depo-medroxyprogesterone acetate subcutaneously. *Contraception.* 2010;81(6):487. doi:10.1016/j.contraception.2010.01.021

12. Cromer BA, Scholes D, Berenson A, Cundy T, Clark MK, Kaunitz AM. Depot medroxyprogesterone acetate and bone mineral density in adolescents—the black box warning: a position paper of the society for adolescent medicine, society for adolescent medicine. *J Adolesc Health.* 2006;39(2):296. doi:10.1016/j.jadohealth.2006.03.011

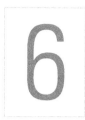

BIRTH CONTROL: SUBDERMAL IMPLANT

Jennifer Kurkowski

INTRODUCTION

The etonogestrel implant is a single-rod progestin-only contraceptive method.[1] The implant is a small 4 cm × 2 mm semi-rigid plastic rod containing 68 mg of the progestin etonogestrel and is radiopaque.[1] The hormone is slowly released over 3 years but recent studies suggest the implant can be used up to 5 years.[2] Fewer than one in 100 women become pregnant while using the implant.[3]

INITIATION

The implant can be inserted at any time during a women's cycle if pregnancy can be reasonably excluded.[1]

COMMON PATIENT CONCERNS

- Changes in menstrual cycle
- Mood changes
- Breast tenderness
- Weight gain
- Medication interactions
- Insertion site concerns

⊙ KEY QUESTIONS TO ASK

Amenorrhea

- Was there any chance of pregnancy prior to the implant insertion?
- Was the patient transitioning from another effective form of birth control prior to insertion? If not, did the patient have unprotected intercourse within 7 days of insertion?
- When was the patient's last menstrual period (LMP)?

Irregular bleeding

- When did the bleeding start?
- How many pads or tampons has the patient been changing? How saturated are the pads or tampons?
- Has the patient had any new sexual partners or is there a potential for exposure to a sexually transmitted infection (STI)?

Postinsertion concerns

- Is the patient experiencing any local side effects such as pain, swelling, bruising, or a hematoma at incision site?
- Is the patient experiencing any neuropathic pain?

Concerns the implant migrated or broke

- How far has the implant migrated?
- Is the patient able to palpate the implant?

Concerns about removal

- Does the patient desire removal?
- Is the patient experiencing any local side effects such as pain, swelling, bruising, or a hematoma?

For backup contraception

- When was the implant placed?
- If inserted recently, was the patient previously using an effective form of birth control?
- Is the patient using any medications?

TABLE 6.1 Patient Assessment for the Contraceptive Implant

Side Effects/Patient Concerns	Counseling /Intervention/Delegation
Medication interactions	- Certain medications can decrease the efficacy of hormonal implants. Patients using any of these medications may need to use a backup method of contraception. - Anticonvulsants: phenytoin, carbamazepine, **barbiturates**, primidone, topiramate, **and** oxcarbazepine. - Certain antiviral drugs used for HIV: **EFV, FPV, and ritonavir-boosted therapies.**

(continued)

TABLE 6.1 Patient Assessment for the Contraceptive Implant (*continued*)

Side Effects/Patient Concerns	Counseling /Intervention/Delegation
	▪ In general, the implant can still be used by patients taking these medications as benefits typically outweigh the risk.[1] ▪ The nurse should consult with a provider regarding any medications the patient may have initiated following the previous office visit.
Amenorrhea	▪ Recommend a pregnancy test if the implant was inserted when pregnancy could not be reasonably excluded and/or if the patient did not follow backup contraception recommendations. ▪ Provide reassurance that is normal for some women to experience amenorrhea while using the implant.[1] ▪ If the patient reports amenorrhea along with severe abdominal pain, see red flag section.
For irregular bleeding	▪ Provide reassurance that most users of the implant will experience changes in their menstrual pattern. This may include amenorrhea, shorter cycles, or longer cycles. ▪ The bleeding pattern may not improve with continued use.[4] ▪ While treatment is not necessary for irregular bleeding, it can be used for patients who are bothered by the unscheduled bleeding. Medications used include NSAIDs, combined oral contraceptive pill.[5] The nurse should consult with a provider to see if treatment is recommended. ▪ Consider STI testing if clinically indicated. ▪ The nurse should recommend an office visit to discuss any bothersome bleeding.
Concerns after insertion	▪ Discuss with the patient that local reactions are rare.[4] ▪ If signs of infection are present, please schedule a clinic visit. ▪ Ulnar nerve damage is a rare but serious side effect. If this is suspected, a clinic visit should be scheduled.[6] See the "red flags" section. ▪ Recommend supportive measures such as warm compresses. ▪ Medications can be used for pain including acetaminophen and NSAIDs.
Concerns about removal	▪ Review with the patient that the implant can be removed at any time if the patient desires.[1] ▪ If signs of an infection are present at the insertion site, please schedule a clinic visit for evaluation.

(*continued*)

TABLE 6.1 Patient Assessment for the Contraceptive Implant (*continued*)

Side Effects/Patient Concerns	Counseling /Intervention/Delegation
	▪ Recommend supportive measures such as warm compresses. ▪ Medications can be used for pain, including acetaminophen and NSAIDs.
For backup contraception	▪ Discuss backup contraception should be used for 7 days after insertion if the implant was inserted >5 days since the beginning of the last menstrual cycle.[2] ▪ Consider emergency contraception if the patient did not follow the backup contraception recommendations
Concerns the implant broke or moved	▪ Review with the patient that it can be normal for the implant to migrate up to 2 cm.[7] ▪ If the implant can no longer be palpated, please schedule a clinic visit. Imaging can be used to localize the implant.[8]

EFV, efavirenz; FPV, fosamprenavir; NSAIDs: nonsteroidal anti-inflammatory drugs; STI, Sexually transmitted infection.

➡ RED FLAGS

Heavy vaginal bleeding: Patients experiencing heavy bleeding associated with symptoms such as shortness of breath, dizziness, lightheadedness, headaches, and syncopal episodes should be referred to the ED for evaluation of symptomatic anemia.

Pelvic pain: Patients who develop significantly worsening pain not improved with nonsteroidal anti-inflammatory drugs (NSAIDs) and/or heating pads should be seen for an urgent evaluation, as this could be a sign of an ectopic pregnancy along with other serious conditions.

Signs of infection: Redness, swelling, severe pain, exudate from insertion site, and/or fever may be concerning for an insertion site infection. If the patient is experiencing these symptoms, a clinical evaluation is warranted. If the patient has access to an online patient portal, the nurse may recommend uploading a picture into the patient portal as well.

Nerve Damage: Nerve damage has been reported in users of the contraceptive implants. Risk factors for this include low body mass index (BMI), migration of the device, or improper insertion.[6] If a patient reports neuropathic pain, surrounding dry erythematous skin, and/or loss of voluntary movement, the patient should be evaluated immediately by a provider.[6]

⊙ SPECIAL POPULATION CONSIDERATIONS

Obese Patients

The implant can be used in obese women as studies have shown no decrease in contraceptive efficacy even though etonogestrel concentration is affected by weight.[9]

Post-abortion

The implant can be immediately inserted after any type of abortion.[1]

Menstrual suppression

There are no contraindications to use the implant in special need patients who desire menstrual suppression, although the amenorrhea can be less compared to other options such as the levonorgestrel intrauterine device.

TABLE 6.2 Commonly Prescribed Medicines for Special Needs Patients With Contraceptive Implants

Medicine	Common Side Effects
Norethindrone	Menstrual irregularities, amenorrhea, nausea
OCPs	Nausea, vomiting, headache
NSAIDs	Nausea, dyspepsia, rash

OCP, oral contraceptive pill; NSAIDs: nonsteroidal anti-inflammatory drugs.

MANAGING SIDE EFFECTS

Consult with a provider if the patient reports any side effects.

SUMMARY

- The contraceptive implant is a highly effective, reversible long-term option for patients in need of contraception.
- The hormone is slowly released over 3 years but recent studies suggest the implant can be used up to 5 years.[2]
- Patients will likely experience menstrual irregularities while having the implant, so effective counseling is important prior to insertion is important.
- The implant can be inserted at any time when a female is not pregnant.
- The implant is a relatively safe contraceptive option in most patients.

RELATED PROTOCOLS

- Chapter 8: Bleeding Concerns
- Chapter 13: Acute Pelvic Pain
- Chapter 14: Chronic Pelvic Pain

References

1. Curtis KM, Tepper NK, Jatlaoui TC, et al. U.S. medical eligibility criteria for contraceptive use, 2016. *MMWR Recomm Rep*. 2016;65(3):1. doi:10.15585/mmwr.rr6503a1
2. McNicholas C, Maddipati R, Zhao Q, Swor E, Peipert JF. Use of the etonogestrel implant and levonorgestrel intrauterine device beyond the U.S. Food and drug administration-approved duration. *Obstet Gynecol*. 2015;125(3):599. doi:10.1097/AOG.0000000000000690
3. Trussell J. Contraceptive failure in the United States. *Contraception*. 2011;83:397–404. doi:10.1016/j.contraception.2011.01.021
4. Nexplanon-etonogestrel implant. US Food and drug administration (FDA) approved product information. US national library of medicine. www.dailymed.nlm.nih.gov; https://dailymed.nlm.nih.gov/dailymed/drugInfo.cfm?setid=b03a3917-9a65-45c2-bbbb-871da858ef34 Accessed May 29, 2019.
5. Guiahi M, McBride M, Sheeder J, Teal S. Short-term treatment of bothersome bleeding for etonogestrel implant users using a 14-day oral contraceptive pill regimen: a randomized controlled trial. *Obstet Gynecol*. 2015;126(3):508–513. doi:10.1097/AOG.0000000000000974
6. O'Grady EE, Power DM. Ulnar nerve injury on removal of a contraceptive implant. *Practitioner*. 2016;260(1799):21.
7. Ismail H, Mansour D, Singh M. Migration of implanon. *J Fam Plann Reprod Health Care*. 2006;32(3):157. doi:10.1783/147118906777888413
8. Gallon A, Fontarensky M, Chauffour C, Boyer L, Chabrot P. Looking for a lost subdermal contraceptive implant? Think about the pulmonary artery. *Contraception*. 2017;95(2):215. doi:10.1016/j.contraception.2016.11.004
9. Morrell KM, Cremers S, Westhoff CL, Davis AR. Relationship between etonogestrel level and BMI in women using the contraceptive implant for more than 1 year. *Contraception*. 2016;93(3):263. doi:10.1016/j.contraception.2015.11.005

7

BIRTH CONTROL: INTRAUTERINE DEVICES

Dana Lenobel

INTRODUCTION

Intrauterine devices (IUDs) are small, T-shaped devices that are placed into the uterine cavity. They are used to help prevent pregnancy and some may also help with menstrual difficulties such as heavy menstrual bleeding or pain. There are two categories of IUDs in the United States: copper-containing IUDs, of which there is one type, and hormonal IUDs that contain the progesterone hormone levonorgestrel, of which there are four types, each releasing a different amount of levonorgestrel and with differing recommended durations of use.

TYPES OF IUDS

Copper IUD: This IUD is a hormone-free IUD that contains 380 mm[1] of copper and is latex free.[2] This IUD is Food and Drug Administration (FDA) approved for 10 years and can also be used as emergency contraception if inserted within 120 hours of unprotected intercourse.[2] It can then be left in place for use.[1] The copper IUD coils prevent sperm from reaching the egg but do not stop ovaries from ovulating each month, therefore cysts may occur, but they usually disappear. Bleeding patterns can be heavier and menses can be longer in length than typical menses.

Hormonal IUDs: Contain as low as 13.5 mg and as high as 52 mg of the progesterone hormone levonorgestrel. The hormonal IUDs last from 3 to 6 years, depending on the IUD. These IUDs prevent pregnancy by thickening the cervical mucus, inhibiting sperm movement, and reducing sperm survival. The Mirena® (levonorgestrel 52 mg; Bayer New Jersey USA) IUD is FDA approved to treat heavy menses because the amount of hormone released inside the uterus keeps the lining thin to decrease bleeding.

CLINICAL PEARL BOX

Noncontraceptive benefits of hormonal IUDs include reduction in heavy bleeding, anemia, dysmenorrhea, endometriosis-related pain, endometrial hyperplasia, pelvic inflammatory disease (PID) risk and risks for cervical cancer.[3-8] All levonorgestrel IUDs also reduce the risk of endometrial and ovarian cancer.[9]

INITIATION

- The IUD can be inserted at any time when pregnancy can be reliably excluded. The provider helps determine the acceptable timing based on the patient's menstrual history and last episode of sexual intercourse.
- If a patient has a known or suspected sexually transmitted infections (STI) and/or symptoms of an active pelvic or vaginal infection, the IUD insertion should be delayed until after the appropriate testing and treatment has been completed.[10]
- Patient may have cramping or pain, bleeding, or dizziness during and right after the procedure.
- Screening for STI should follow current guidelines and can be performed prior to insertion.

REMOVALS

- The IUD must be removed anywhere from 3 to 12 years depending on which type of IUD the patient has in place. Another IUD may be replaced at the time of removal.
- The IUD may be removed at any time during the menstrual cycle and is typically faster and less painful than the IUD insertion.
- Patients should never try to remove the IUD themselves at home.
- Once the IUD is removed, the patient no longer has birth control.
- It can take up to 3 months after IUD removal for the patient's normal menstrual cycle to return.
- The patient may have slight cramping and some light bleeding several hours to several days after IUD removal.

COMMON PATIENT CONCERNS

- Amenorrhea
- Unscheduled bleeding or spotting
- Missing or shortened IUD strings
- Pelvic pain or cramping

⊙ KEY QUESTIONS TO ASK

Amenorrhea

- Is the patient sexually active? Have they taken a home pregnancy test?
- Which IUD do they have in place?
- When did they have the IUD placed?

Unscheduled bleeding or spotting

- When was the IUD inserted and what kind of IUD do they have?
- Any associated pelvic pain?
- Has the patient had unprotected sex, which might indicate an STI or pregnancy?
- Can the patient feel the IUD strings?
- When did the bleeding start?
- How many pads or tampons has the patient been changing? How saturated are the pads or tampons?

Strings concerns

- When was the last time the patient felt the IUD strings?
- If they are sexually active, can their partner feel the IUD strings?
- Are they having trouble locating their strings?
- Any associated pelvic or abdominal pain?

Pelvic pain or cramping

- When did the pelvic pain start?
- How would the patient rate their pain on a scale 1 to 10 in severity?
- Any exacerbating or alleviating factors?
- Any urinary or bowel complaints?
- Any bleeding or vaginal discharge/odor/itching with the pelvic pain?
- Have they tried any over the counter medication or heating pads to help improve their pain?
- When was the IUD placed?

ACUTE/CHRONIC CONCERNS

TABLE 7.1 Acute/Chronic Concerns for the Intrauterine Device

Patient Concerns	Counseling/Interventions
Amenorrhea	■ Some of the IUDs cause amenorrhea and may be the desired effect. The patient should be reassured that this is a common side effect.

(continued)

TABLE 7.1 Acute/Chronic Concerns for the Intrauterine Device (*continued*)

Patient Concerns	Counseling/Interventions
	■ If the patient is sexually active and has any concerns about possible pregnancy, an at-home pregnancy test should be performed.
	■ If the patient has a positive pregnancy test with the IUD in place, they should be seen in clinic immediately as they may be at a higher risk of ectopic pregnancy.[2]
Bleeding or spotting	■ Breakthrough bleeding and irregular bleeding is one of the most common patient complaints within the first few months after IUD insertion.
	■ Bleeding with hormonal IUDs should typically resolve with time, and patients may develop amenorrhea.
	■ Unscheduled bleeding or spotting can also be a sign of STI or a vaginal infection. If the patient has been sexually active and has not had recent STI testing or vaginal testing, offer/recommend an appointment. If they are positive for an STI or vaginal infection, the IUD may stay in place.[10]
	■ For any heavy or prolonged bleeding please see chapter on heavy vaginal bleeding or additional assessment questions/management.
	■ The triage nurse should ask the patient if they can feel their strings. If they cannot feel their strings they need an office visit to check for placement. Bleeding could be due to the IUD being in the wrong position.
	■ If a patient has ongoing heavy and/or prolonged bleeding, they need an exam to exclude IUD malposition or expulsion, pregnancy, or infection.[11]
	■ Medical treatment should be considered for women who continue to have bothersome bleeding up to 3 months from IUD insertion.
Pelvic pain, cramping	■ Discuss NSAIDs and heating pads as needed for discomfort.
	■ Patients who develop significantly worsening pain not improved with NSAIDs and/or heating pads should be seen for an urgent evaluation, as this could be a sign of an IUD complication or infection.
	■ Ask the patient if she has urinary, bowel, musculoskeletal, or severe psychosocial complaints. These additional complaints could be the reasons for the pelvic pain and can be evaluated at an office visit.
String concerns	■ If the patient cannot feel their strings the nurse should recommend an office visit.
	■ The patient should refrain from intercourse or use another contraceptive method until the IUD is confirmed as in the correct position.

(*continued*)

TABLE 7.1 Acute/Chronic Concerns for the Intrauterine Device (*continued*)

Patient Concerns	Counseling/Interventions
	▪ If the **strings are visible on exam** but not felt by the patient: The strings can curl up into the cervix but still be in the correct position or sometimes the patient's fingers are not long enough to reach the strings.
	▪ If **strings are not visible on exam** and unable to be retrieved by the provider: This frequently means that the strings are in the cervical os. The patient should see and discuss with their provider to confirm placement.
	▪ If the **strings are not visible on exam** however in the correct position on imaging: The IUD can be left in place.
	▪ If the **strings are not visible on exam and the IUD is not visible on a pelvic ultrasound**, a KUB should be completed to determine if the IUD was expulsed or if it is in the abdominal cavity.
	▪ If a partner can feel the strings during intercourse and it is causing pain, then the strings should be trimmed in the office.
	▪ Women are no longer routinely recommended to check their strings. There is no evidence to support this practice.[12,13]

KUB, kidney ureter and bladder x-ray; NSAIDs, nonsteroid anti-inflammatory agent; STI, sexually transmitted infection.

➡ RED FLAGS

▪ **Heavy vaginal bleeding:** Patients experiencing heavy bleeding associated with symptoms such as shortness of breath, dizziness, lightheadedness, headaches, and syncopal episodes should be referred to the ED for evaluation of symptomatic anemia.

▪ **Pelvic pain:** Patients who develop significantly worsening pain not improved with nonsteroid anti-inflammatory agents (NSAIDs) and/or heating pads should be seen for an urgent evaluation, as this could be a sign of an IUD complication or infection.

⊙ SPECIAL POPULATION CONSIDERATIONS

The IUD is generally safe for the majority of young females. In most cases, the IUD should not be inserted in premenarchal patients but can be initiated once menarche is achieved. The IUD can be placed with the assistance of anxiolytics or general anesthesia.

Some of the reasons that represent an unacceptable health risk (contraindication) to an IUD insertion include[14-17]

- Active STI
- Acute pelvic Iiflammatory disease
- Acute liver disease or liver carcinoma (levonorgestrel IUD)
- Breast carcinoma (levonorgestrel IUD)
- Confirmed or suspected pregnancy
- Copper allergy (copper IUD)
- Genital actinomycosis
- Jaundice (levonorgestrel IUD)
- Known or suspected pelvic malignancy
- Postpartum endometritis or septic abortion in previous 3 months
- Undiagnosed vaginal bleeding
- Uterine abnormality
- Wilson's disease (copper IUD)

Patients with developmental delay: IUDs may be inserted in the operating room or special exam room with sedation if an in-office procedure is not expected to be tolerated.

Patients with heavy menstrual bleeding: Some hormonal IUDs are FDA approved for patients with heavy menstrual bleeding and are therefore considered an excellent option for this population and for patients where menstrual suppression is desired.

Patients with a known or suspected bleeding disorder: Patients with a known or suspected bleeding disorder may be at higher risk for bleeding complications with any procedure. The patient's gynecology provider will need to consult with the patient's hematologist prior to the IUD insertion to determine if additional measures and/or medications need to be utilized for the procedure.

Nulliparous patients: Any IUD is considered safe (given no contraindications) if a patient has never delivered a baby. The uterine length is important to know because the minimum uterine size for both the levonorgestrel 52 mcg IUD and copper IUD is 6 cm. There is not a minimum uterus size for the smaller IUDs.

Patients who are not sexually active: Patients can have the IUD placed (given no contraindications) regardless of sexual activity. The patient's provider may recommend a trial with a speculum exam before considering an IUD insertion in the office. If a patient is extremely anxious or not cooperative for a speculum exam, an IUD under sedation is a good option.

SUMMARY

- IUDs are a top tier option for adolescents who desire a highly effective, long-acting, reversible contraception method. It is an ideal method for patients who need to avoid estrogen (all IUDs) or all hormonal exposure (copper IUD).

- Serious IUD complications are uncommon but include expulsion, contraceptive failure, and perforation.
- Less serious side effects include malposition, pain, and irregular bleeding patterns.
- Side effects that commonly occur in the first week following insertion include bleeding and uterine cramping. The cramping frequently abates quickly, but bleeding can take a few months for most.

RELATED PROTOCOLS

- Chapter 10: Dysmenorrhea
- Chapter 8: Abnormal uterine bleeding
- CDC contraceptive guidelines

References

1. Cleland K, Raymond EG, Westley E, Trussell J. Emergency contraception review: evidence-based recommendations for clinicians. *Clin Obstet Gynecol.* 2014;57:741. doi:10.1097/GRF.0000000000000056
2. ParaGard [package insert]. Tonawanda, NY: FEI Products, 2003.
3. Cortessis VK, Barrett M, Brown Wade N, et al. Intrauterine device use and cervical cancer risk: a systematic review and meta-analysis. *Obstet Gynecol.* 2017;130:1226. doi:10.1097/AOG.0000000000002307
4. Abou-Setta AM, Al-Inany HG, Farquhar CM. Levonorgestrel-releasing intrauterine device (LNG-IUD) for symptomatic endometriosis following surgery. *Cochrane Database Syst Rev.* 2006;(4):CD005072. doi:10.1002/14651858.CD005072.pub2
5. Lethaby AE, Cooke I, Rees M. Progesterone or progestogen-releasing intrauterine systems for heavy menstrual bleeding. *Cochrane Database Syst Rev.* 2005; CD002126. doi:10.1002/14651858.CD002126.pub2
6. Cim N, Soysal S, Sayan S, et al. Two years follow-up of patients with abnormal uterine bleeding after insertion of the levonorgestrel-releasing intrauterine system. *Gynecol Obstet Invest.* 2018;83:569. doi:10.1159/000480012
7. Kaunitz AM, Bissonnette F, Monteiro I, et al. Levonorgestrel-releasing intrauterine system or medroxyprogesterone for heavy menstrual bleeding: a randomized controlled trial. *Obstet Gynecol.* 2010;116:625. doi:10.1097/AOG.0b013e3181ec622b
8. Baker WD, Pierce SR, Mills AM, et al. Nonoperative management of atypical endometrial hyperplasia and grade 1 endometrial cancer with the levonorgestrel intrauterine device in medically ill post-menopausal women. *Gynecol Oncol.* 2017;146:34. doi:10.1016/j.ygyno.2017.04.006
9. Madden, T. Intrauterine contraception: background and device types. *UpToDate.* July 1, 2019. https://www.uptodate.com/contents/intrauterine-contraception -background-and-device-types?search=iud&source=search_result&selectedTitle= 1~150&usage_type=default&display_rank=1
10. Workowski KA, Bolan GA, Centers for Disease Control and Prevention. Sexually transmitted diseases treatment guidelines, 2015. *MMWR Recomm Rep.* 2015;64:1.

11. Pocius KD, Bartz DA. Intrauterine contraception: management of side effects and complications. *UpToDate*. July 1, 2019. https://www.uptodate.com/contents/intrauterine-contraception-management-of-side-effects-and complications?search=iud&source=search_result&selectedTitle=2~150&usage_type=default&display_rank=2

12. Curtis KM, Jatlaoui TC, Tepper NK, et al. U.S. Selected practice recommendations for contraceptive use, 2016. *MMWR Recomm Rep*. 2016;65:1. doi:10.15585/mmwr.rr6504a1

13. Melo J, Tschann M, Soon R, et al. Women's willingness and ability to feel the strings of their intrauterine device. *Int J Gynaecol Obstet*. 2017;137:309. doi:10.1002/ijgo.12130

14. *Mirena [Package insert]*. Montville, NJ: Berlex Laboratories, 2003.

15. Nelson AL. The intrauterine contraceptive device. *Obstet Gynecol Clin North Am*. 2000;27:723–740. doi:10.1016/S0889-8545(05)70170-4

16. Canavan TP. Appropriate use of the intrauterine device. *Am Fam Physician*. 1998;58:2077–2084, 2087–2088.

17. Johnson BA. Insertion and removal of intrauterine devices. 2005. https://www.aafp.org/afp/2005/0101/p95.html

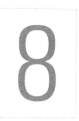

8

BLEEDING CONCERNS
Jane Geyer

INTRODUCTION

Abnormal uterine bleeding (AUB) is one of the most common patient concerns in the adolescent population. AUB is defined by menstrual bleeding that occurs outside of the normal range and can include irregular bleeding patterns; prolonged or short bleeding episodes; and heavy or light bleeding.[1] In the adolescent population, AUB is most commonly due to anovulatory cycles, which may occur during the first few years after the patient's first menstrual period (menarche) as a result of an immature hypothalamic-pituitary-ovarian axis.[2,3] Nonetheless, AUB almost always warrants an evaluation, whether emergently for acute bleeding episodes or routinely during an office visit for chronic and/or stable AUB.

In order to determine abnormal bleeding amounts and/or patterns, it is important to understand the normal parameters for a menstrual cycle in this age group. Although menstrual cycles can significantly vary in the first several years following menarche, most adolescents have a menstrual period every 21 to 45 days and bleed for 3 to 7 days.[4,5] Cycle patterns and length of periods typically become more regular as patients progress through puberty.[5] The amount of blood loss can be difficult to determine due to the vast amount of hygiene products on the market and perception bias between each patient.[6-8] The patient should note how many products she is changing on average and estimate how saturated each product is.[9]

Nurses and healthcare providers must collect as much information as possible about the menstrual bleeding to help determine the appropriate plan of care.

COMMON PATIENT CONCERNS

- Heavy menstrual bleeding
- Irregular bleeding patterns
- Prolonged menstrual bleeding
- Intermenstrual bleeding or spotting

(O) KEY QUESTIONS TO ASK

Heavy menstrual bleeding

- Is the patient experiencing signs and symptoms of anemia, such as feeling light-headed, dizzy, short of breath, or lethargic? Is the patient experiencing pallor?
- Is the patient sexually active, and if so, is there any chance of pregnancy?
- When did the bleeding start?
- How many pads or tampons has the patient been changing per day?
- How saturated are the pads (e.g., < 25%, 25%–50%, 50%–100%, or overflowing)?
- Is the patient passing blood clots? If so, how large are the clots?

Irregular menstrual bleeding

- When was the patient's last menstrual period (LMP)?
- Has the patient been keeping a menstrual calendar? If so, inquire about the patient's cycle patterns in the last 6 to 12 months.
- How many days do the patient's cycles typically last?
- How many pads or tampons does the patient change per day?
- How saturated are the pads/tampons?
- Is the patient sexually active, and if so, is there any chance of pregnancy?

Prolonged menstrual bleeding

- Is the patient experiencing signs and symptoms of anemia, such as feeling light-headed, dizzy, short of breath, or lethargic? Is the patient experiencing pallor?
- Is the patient sexually active, and if so, is there any chance of pregnancy?
- When did the bleeding start?
- How many pads or tampons has the patient been changing per day?
- How saturated are the patient's pads (e.g., < 25%, 25%–50%, 50%–100%, or overflowing)?
- Is the patient passing blood clots? If so, how large are the clots?

Intermenstrual bleeding

- When was the patient's most recent LMP?
- How often does the patient normally have a menstrual cycle?
- Is the patient sexually active? If so, has the patient had unprotected intercourse?
- Is the patient experiencing any pelvic/abdominal pain associated with the bleeding?
- Is the patient experiencing vaginal symptoms such as discharge?
- Is the patient using hormonal contraception? If so, please proceed to the appropriate chapter for additional triage questions/management.

CLINICAL PEARL BOX

The nurse should recommend the patient download a menstrual cycle application to help track menstrual cycles and heaviness of flow.

TABLE 8.1 Acute Symptoms of Abnormal Uterine Bleeding

Acute Symptoms	Interventions/Counseling	Commonly Prescribed Medications
HMB	■ For any signs/symptoms of hemodynamic instability, the patient should be instructed to go to the ED. If the patient is not symptomatic, arrange an urgent office visit. ■ If there is any chance of pregnancy, the patient should be instructed to go to the ED ■ If the patient is saturating a pad every 1–2 hours, the patient should be instructed to go to the ED.	■ Hormonal contraceptive options ■ Tranexamic acid ■ Desmopressin ■ Aminocaproic Acid
Prolonged menstrual bleeding	■ For any signs/symptoms of hemodynamic instability, the patient should be instructed to go to the ED. If the patient is not symptomatic, arrange an urgent office visit. ■ If there is any chance of pregnancy, the patient should be instructed to go to the ED. ■ If the patient is saturating a pad every 1–2 hours, the patient should be instructed to go to the ED.	■ Hormonal contraceptive options ■ Tranexamic acid ■ Desmopressin ■ Aminocaproic Acid
Intermenstrual bleeding	■ If the patient is sexually active, recommend an at-home UPT. ■ If the patient has any associated pelvic/abdominal pain, please notify a provider. This may warrant a same-day visit and/or ED visit.	■ Hormonal contraception ■ Azithromycin with or without ceftriaxone in case of cervical infection

(continued)

TABLE 8.1 Acute Symptoms of Abnormal Uterine Bleeding (*continued*)

Acute Symptoms	Interventions/Counseling	Commonly Prescribed Medications
	▧ If the patient is on hormonal contraception and experiencing breakthrough bleeding, please proceed to associated chapter for management.	

HMB, heavy menstrual bleeding; UPT, urine pregnancy test.

TABLE 8.2 Chronic Symptoms of Abnormal Uterine Bleeding

Chronic Symptoms		Common Medications Prescribed
Heavy menstrual bleeding	▧ This may be due to a multitude of underlying conditions, such as bleeding disorders or thyroid abnormalities, or anovulatory in nature due to hormonal imbalances or recent menarche. ▧ A clinical evaluation is always indicated. ▧ The nurse should review all triage questions to assess for changes and red flags. ▧ The nurse should document which medications the patient has been taking for the provider to review. ▧ The nurse should recommend the patient keep a menstrual calendar to bring to next visit.	▧ Hormonal contraceptives ▧ Tranexamic acid ▧ Aminocaproic Acid ▧ Desmopressin
Prolonged menstrual periods	▧ This may be due to a multitude of underlying conditions, such as bleeding disorders, thyroid abnormalities, or infections, or anovulatory in nature due to hormonal imbalances or recent menarche.	▧ Hormonal contraceptives ▧ Tranexamic acid ▧ Aminocaproic Acid ▧ Desmopressin

(*continued*)

TABLE 8.2 Chronic Symptoms of Abnormal Uterine Bleeding (*continued*)

Chronic Symptoms		Common Medications Prescribed
	▪ A clinical evaluation is always indicated. ▪ The nurse should review all triage questions to assess for changes and red flags. ▪ The nurse should document which medications the patient has been taking for the provider to review. ▪ The nurse should recommend the patient keep a menstrual calendar to bring to next visit.	
Frequent menstrual cycles	▪ This may be due to a multitude of underlying conditions such as bleeding disorders, thyroid abnormalities, infections, or hormonal imbalances. ▪ A clinical evaluation is always indicated. ▪ The nurse should review all triage questions to assess for changes and red flags. ▪ The nurse should document which medications the patient has been taking for the provider to review. ▪ The nurse should recommend the patient keep a menstrual calendar to bring to next visit.	▪ Hormonal contraceptives ▪ Tranexamic acid ▪ Aminocaproic Acid ▪ Desmopressin
Intermenstrual spotting	▪ This may be anovulatory in nature and a clinical evaluation is usually indicated. ▪ If this occurs solely after intercourse or sexual activity, it may indicate a cervical/vaginal infection, and a clinical evaluation is indicated.	▪ Hormonal contraceptives

(*continued*)

TABLE 8.2 Chronic Symptoms of Abnormal Uterine Bleeding (*continued*)

Chronic Symptoms		Common Medications Prescribed
	▪ If the patient is on hormonal contraception and experiencing breakthrough bleeding, please proceed to associated chapter for management. ▪ The nurse should recommend the patient keep a menstrual calendar to bring to next visit.	

➡ RED FLAGS

For any AUB concerns, the nurse should first assess for hemodynamic instability and if there is a chance of pregnancy.

▪ **Acute symptomatic anemia:**
- Symptoms may include lethargy, dizziness, shortness of breath at rest or with mild exertion, fatigue. In extreme cases of anemia, patients may experience chest pain, arrhythmias.
- Severe anemia from blood loss can be life-threatening. Patients experiencing symptoms should always be sent to the ED.

▪ **Pregnancy:**
- Bleeding during pregnancy can be physiologic or can be a sign of ectopic pregnancy, spontaneous abortion, gestational trophoblastic concern, or a vaginal/uterine pathology.
- Physiologic bleeding in those with known or suspected pregnancy is a diagnosis of exclusion, therefore the triage nurse should notify a provider immediately and refer the patient to the ED for assessment.

⊙ SPECIAL POPULATION CONSIDERATIONS

Bleeding and coagulation disorders: Up to 20% of females with heavy menstrual bleeding or significant AUB have an underlying bleeding disorder.[10] Bleeding disorders may include Von Willebrand disease, factor deficiencies, and platelet dysfunction. These patients may be at higher risk for excessive blood loss and anemia.

TABLE 8.3 Commonly Prescribed Medicines for Treatment of Abnormal Uterine Bleeding

Medication	Side Effects/ Counseling*	Interactions
Combination hormonal therapy (OCPs) Often prescribed as a taper for acute management, which initially begins with much higher doses of estrogen. Once stabilized, patients typically switch to continuous or regular cyclic regimens of OCPs.	**See OCP chapter** Side effects may be amplified on the higher doses of OCPs compared with traditional pill doses. Consult with a provider for any side effects a patient experiences while using a hormonal taper.	**See OCP chapter**
Hormonal contraception All options may be utilized to help management AUB.	**See each individual chapter for side effects**	**See each individual chapter for interactions**
Norethindrone Acetate Often given as a taper: 1 tab BID × 7 days, then 1 tab daily × 7 days	Breast tenderness Acne Weight gain Mood changes[11]	Ulipristal (avoid use of progestins within 5 days of use)[11] Consult with a provider for additional medication interactions.
Medroxyprogesterone May be given as PO taper or IM or SQ injection	Breast tenderness Weight gain (more common with IM).[12]	Ulipristal (avoid use of progestins within 5 days of use)[12] Consult with a provider for additional medication interactions.
Tranexamic acid[2] Dosing: 1,300 mg TID × up to 5 days each month	Headaches Fatigue Abdominal pain Muscle pain/spasms Vision changes Seizures VTE[13] Consult with a GYN or hematology provider if the patient is experiencing side effects.	Avoid use with anti-inhibitor coagulant complex (Human). May increase thrombotic effects in patients using hormonal contraceptives.[13]

(continued)

TABLE 8.3 Commonly Prescribed Medicines for Treatment of Abnormal Uterine Bleeding (*continued*)

Medication	Side Effects/ Counseling*	Interactions
Aminocaproic acid Consult with hematology provider/prescriber regarding dose	Dizziness Headaches Weakness Diarrhea, cramps, nausea/vomiting Cardiac changes and/or arrhythmias Blood pressure changes[14] Consult with a GYN or hematology provider if the patient is experiencing any side effects with this medication.	Avoid use with anti-inhibitor coagulant complex (Human) and Factor IX Complex (Human Factors II, IX, X). Avoid use in patients with renal impairment.[14] Consult with hematologist for additional interactions.
Desmopressin Consult with hematology provider/prescriber regarding dose	Dry mouth Hyponatremia Headache/dizziness Abdominal pain Nausea[15] Consult with a GYN or hematology provider if the patient is experiencing side effects.	Avoid excessive fluid intake with this medication. Avoid taking with loop diuretics, corticosteroids, NSAIDs, SSRIs, or tolvaptan.[15] Consult with a hematologist for additional interactions.
Ferrous Sulfate Dosage: 325 mg ferrous sulfate (elemental iron 65 mg) Often taken: once daily or BID.	Constipation Abdominal pain Darkening of stools Nausea/vomiting Take with juice or on an empty stomach. Can administer with food to help prevent gastrointestinal (GI) upset. Avoid consuming with cereals, teas, coffee, or milk.[16] Consult with a GYN or hematology provider if the patient is experiencing side effects.	Avoid use with antacids as this can cause decreased iron absorption. Avoid taking concurrently with cefdinir, tetracyclines, levothyroxine, or quniolones. Consult with provider for how to time ferrous sulfate dosing when using the above medications.[16] Consult with a provider for additional interactions.

AUB, abnormal uterine bleeding; NSAIDs, nonsteroidal anti-inflammatory drugs; OCPs, oral contraceptive pills; VTE, venous thromboembolism; SSRIs, selective serotonin reuptake inhibitors.

*The nurse should consult with a provider regarding any side effects a patient may experience.

SUMMARY

▪ AUB is defined by menstrual bleeding that occurs outside of the normal range and can include irregular bleeding patterns; prolonged or short bleeding episodes; and heavy or light bleeding.[1]

▪ Although menstrual cycles can significantly vary in the first several years following menarche, most adolescents have a menstrual period every 21 to 45 days and bleed for 3 to 7 days.[4,5]

▪ Nurses and healthcare providers must collect as much information about the menstrual bleeding to help determine the appropriate plan of care.

▪ For any AUB concerns, the nurse should first assess for hemodynamic instability and if there is a chance of pregnancy. These patients should always be referred to the ED.

RELATED PROTOCOLS

▪ Menstrual calendars
▪ Pictorial Blood Loss Assessment Chart (PBAC) scores
▪ Hormonal contraceptive chapters (see Chapters 2–7)

References

1. ACOG committee opinion no. 651: menstruation in girls and adolescents: using the menstrual cycle as a vital sign. *Obstet Gynecol*. 2015;126(6):e143. doi:10.1097/AOG.0000000000001215

2. Gunn HM, Tsai MC, McRae A, Steinbeck KS. Menstrual patterns in the first gynecologic year: a systematic review. *J Pediatr Adolesc Gynecol*. 2018;31(6):557–565.e6. Epub 2018 Jul 29.

3. Lemarchand-Béraud T, Zufferey MM, Reymond M, Rey I. Maturation of the hypothalamo-pituitary-ovarian axis in adolescent girls. *J Clin Endocrinol Metab*. 1982;54(2):241. doi:10.1210/jcem-54-2-241

4. Adams Hillard PJ. Menstruation in young girls: a clinical perspective. *Obstet Gynecol*. 2002;99(4):655. doi:10.1016/S0029-7844(02)01660-5

5. Flug D, Largo R, Prader A. Menstrual patterns in adolescent Swiss girls: a longitudinal study. *Ann Hum Biol*. 1984;11(6):495. doi:10.1080/03014468400007411

6. Hallberg L, Högdahl AM, Nilsson L, Rybo G. Menstrual blood loss—a population study. Variation at different ages and attempts to define normality. *Acta Obstet Gynecol Scand*. 1966;45(3):320. doi:10.3109/00016346609158455

7. Reid PC, Coker A, Coltart R. Assessment of menstrual blood loss using a pictorial chart: a validation study. *BJOG*. 2000;107(3):320. doi:10.1111/j.1471-0528.2000.tb13225.x

8. Fraser IS, McCarron G, Markham R. A preliminary study of factors influencing perception of menstrual blood loss volume. *Am J Obstet Gynecol*. 1984;149(7):788. doi:10.1016/0002-9378(84)90123-6

9. Janssen CA, Scholten PC, Heintz AP. A simple visual assessment technique to discriminate between menorrhagia and normal menstrual blood loss. *Obstet Gynecol*. 1995;85(6):977. doi:10.1016/0029-7844(95)00062-V

10. Ahuja S, Hertweck S. Overview of bleeding disorders in adolescent females with menorrhagia. *J Pediatrc Adolesc Gynecol*. 2010;23(Suppl. 6):S15–S21. doi:10.1016/j.jpag.2010.08.006

11. Norethindrone. *Lexi-drugs. Lexicomp.* Riverwoods, IL: Wolters Kluwer Health Inc. http://online.lexi.com. Accessed June 29, 2010.
12. Medroxyprogesterone. *Lexi-drugs. Lexicomp.* Riverwoods, IL: Wolters Kluwer Health Inc. http://online.lexi.com. Accessed June 29, 2010.
13. Tranexamic Acid. *Lexi-drugs. Lexicomp.* Riverwoods, IL: Wolters Kluwer Health Inc. http://online.lexi.com. Accessed June 29, 2010.
14. Aminocaproic acid. *Lexi-drugs. Lexicomp.* Riverwoods, IL: Wolters Kluwer Health Inc. http://online.lexi.com. Accessed June 29, 2010.
15. Vasopressin. *Lexi-drugs. Lexicomp.* Riverwoods, IL: Wolters Kluwer Health Inc. http://online.lexi.com. Accessed June 29, 2010.
16. Ferrous sulfate. *Lexi-drugs. Lexicomp.* Riverwoods, IL: Wolters Kluwer Health Inc. http://online.lexi.com. Accessed June 29, 2010.

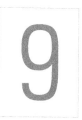

9

BREAST CONCERNS
Jane Geyer

INTRODUCTION

Breast development (thelarche) begins in early puberty and is stimulated by estrogen and progesterone. The average age for thelarche is 10.3 and thelarche typically begins between ages 10 to 13.[1,2] Breast development is an important indicator of pubertal progression, therefore patients who may report early or delayed breast development should always evaluated in the office.

Breast self-awareness is encouraged during adolescent years; however, routine breast examinations are not typically recommended in this population.[3] Most breast abnormalities, including masses, are typically benign in the young population. Nonetheless, these concerns can often be distressing and worrisome to patients and caregivers.

CLINICAL PEARL BOX

Breast self-awareness is encouraged during adolescent years; however, routine breast examinations are not typically recommended in this population.[3]

COMMON PATIENT CONCERNS

- Breast asymmetry
- Breast pain
- Breast lump/mass
- Breast discharge

KEY QUESTIONS TO ASK

Breast asymmetry
- When was this first noted?
- Any trauma to the area?
- Any palpable masses?

Breast pain

- When did the pain start?
- Is the pain localized or generalized?
- Is the pain bilateral or unilateral?
- Are there systemic or other local symptoms present (such as fever or erythema)?
- Are there any palpable abnormalities present (lumps/masses, bump)?
- Has the pain been recurring? If so, has the patient noticed any cyclic breast pain, specifically in relation to menstrual cycles?
- Is there any chance of pregnancy?
- Is the patient using birth control such as oral contraceptive pills (OCPs) or the arm implant?
- Does the patient drink caffeine?
- Does the patient use illicit substances such as marijuana?
- Has the patient recently engaged in any vigorous physical activity?
- Has any trauma or blunt force to the area occurred?

Breast lump/mass

- When was the lump first noted?
- Can the patient describe the lump? (size, shape, mobile versus nonmobile)
- Are there systemic or other local symptoms present (such as fever or erythema)?

Nipple discharge

- When did it start?
- Is the discharge bilateral or unilateral?
- What is the color and consistency of the discharge? (e.g., milky, purulent, blood-tinged, etc.)
- Is the discharge spontaneous or elicited by stimulation of the breast?
- Is the patient sexually active, and if so, is there any chance of pregnancy?
- Has the patient started any new medications recently?
- Are there systemic or other local symptoms present (such as fever or erythema)? Does the patient have a piercing or recent trauma to the area?

TABLE 9.1 Acute Symptoms of Breast Conditions in Adolescents

Acute Symptoms	Counseling/Intervention	Medications Prescribed
Breast pain	■ Recommend well-supportive bras, especially in those with large breasts. Some studies have shown an improvement in breast pain when sports bras	Tylenol or NSAIDs[8]

(continued)

TABLE 9.1 Acute Symptoms of Breast Conditions in Adolescents (*continued*)

Acute Symptoms	Counseling/Intervention	Medications Prescribed
	are worn during physical activity to help prevent the stretching of ligaments between skin and pectoral fascia.[4] ▪ Recommend application of warm compresses to the area. ▪ Recommend avoiding caffeine. Although studies show weak evidence behind this, some patients have reported an improvement in nodular changes and breast pain.[5,6] ▪ Recommend the patient take a home pregnancy test if there is any risk of pregnancy. ▪ Recommend cessation of illicit substances such as marijuana, as this can worsen breast pain.[7] ▪ Recommend a clinic evaluation for assessment.	
Nipple discharge	▪ Provide reassurance that most nipple discharge in children and adolescents is associated with benign causes. ▪ Recommend patient avoid breast stimulation. ▪ Recommend a home pregnancy test if there is any risk of pregnancy. ▪ Recommend a clinical evaluation. ▪ Recommend patient bring a list of medications to the office visit. Certain medications, such as psychotropic and anticonvulsant medications, can elevate prolactin levels.[9]	▪ Antibiotics may be prescribed when breast discharge is caused by an infection.
Breast infection (mastitis)	▪ Rare in nonbreastfeeding women. ▪ In nonbreastfeeding adolescents, infections are typically caused by the introduction of bacteria into the ductal system.[10] ▪ Some risk factors include plucking or shaving hair, piercings, and stimulation during sexual activity.[11]	▪ Antibiotics are indicated for treatment of an infection.

(*continued*)

TABLE 9.1 Acute Symptoms of Breast Conditions in Adolescents (*continued*)

Acute Symptoms	Counseling/Intervention	Medications Prescribed
	▪ Symptoms include fevers/chills and breast warmth, redness, and pain. ▪ Recommend warm compresses and NSAIDs for symptom relief. ▪ Recommend urgent office visit. If this is associated with any systemic symptoms, recommend the patient go to the ED.	
Breast lump/mass	▪ Recommend self-breast examinations to monitor for changes prior to the office visit. ▪ Provide reassurance that most breast lumps are benign in young females.[12] ▪ Recommend clinical evaluation to have the lump assessed. ▪ If systemic symptoms (fevers, chills, pain) are present with the rapid onset of a breast mass, recommend a same-day visit for evaluation. If a clinic visit is not available, recommend that the patient go to the ED.	▪ Antibiotics are prescribed for infectious breast abscesses.

NSAIDs, nonsteroidal anti-inflammatory drugs.

TABLE 9.2 Chronic Symptoms of Breast Conditions in Adolescents

Chronic Symptoms	Counseling/Intervention	Medications Prescribed
Breast asymmetry	▪ Breast asymmetry is common in females and is most pronounced during puberty.[13] ▪ The asymmetry may be more evident in patients with a history of scoliosis, chest wall trauma, and/or infection.[7] ▪ The nurse should recommend an office evaluation for a breast exam to rule out abnormalities and provide reassurance to the family. ▪ A noninvasive intervention may include padded bras. The patient may consider a mastectomy bra/insert that contains more padding on the side of the smaller breast.[14]	▪ Medications are not prescribed for breast asymmetry.

(*continued*)

TABLE 9.2 Chronic Symptoms of Breast Conditions in Adolescents (*continued*)

Chronic Symptoms	Counseling/Intervention	Medications Prescribed
Cyclic breast pain	▪ Recommend well-supportive bras, especially for those with large breasts. Some studies have shown an improvement in breast pain when sports bras are worn during physical activity to help prevent the stretching of ligaments between skin and pectoral fascia.[4] ▪ Recommend application of warm compresses to the area. ▪ Recommend avoiding caffeine. Although studies show weak evidence behind this, some patients have reported an improvement in nodular changes and breast pain.[5,6] ▪ Recommend the patient take an at-home pregnancy test if there is any risk of pregnancy. ▪ Recommend cessation of illicit substances such as marijuana, as this can worsen breast pain.[7] ▪ Recommend a clinic evaluation.	▪ NSAIDs (ibuprofen) ▪ Oral contraceptive pills
Recurrent breast lumps	▪ Most lumps that are recurrent and self-resolving are fibrocystic breast changes, especially if symptoms begin prior to menstruation and resolve after menses. ▪ The exact incidence in adolescents is unknown, but it is estimated that 50% of females of reproductive age experience this.[15] ▪ The nurse should recommend a clinic evaluation for any persistent breast lumps. ▪ A breast ultrasound may be warranted. Instruct the patient to perform self-breast exams to monitor for any changes related to the lump(s).	▪ NSAIDs ▪ Oral contraceptive pills

(*continued*)

TABLE 9.2 Chronic Symptoms of Breast Conditions in Adolescents (*continued*)

Chronic Symptoms	Counseling/Intervention	Medications Prescribed
Nipple discharge	▪ Provide reassurance that most nipple discharge in children and adolescents is associated with benign causes. ▪ Recommend patient avoid breast stimulation. ▪ Recommend an at-home pregnancy test if there is any risk of pregnancy. ▪ Recommend a clinical evaluation. ▪ Recommend patient bring a list of medications to the office visit. Certain medications, such as psychotropic and anticonvulsant medications, can elevate prolactin levels.[9]	Medications are not commonly prescribed for chronic nipple discharge in young females.

NSAIDs, nonsteroidal anti-inflammatory drugs.

➡ RED FLAGS

Mastitis: Although mastitis (infection of the breast) is rare in nonbreastfeeding women, it should be considered in patients who report rapid onset of swelling, erythema, warmth, tenderness, and induration.[16,17] Patients who report a breast mass and have associated systemic symptoms (such as fever, malaise), have rapid progression of erythema, or are immunocompromised should be instructed to go to the ED for evaluation.

Ⓞ SPECIAL POPULATIONS TO CONSIDER

- **Cancer patients/patients exposed to radiation:** Exposure to radiation and childhood cancers are both considered risk factors for secondary malignancy in the breast.[18] Imaging is recommended for this population with MRI either 8 years after the treatment occurred, **or** at age 25, depending on whichever occurs last.[19] Hodgkin's lymphoma patients/survivors are at highest risk of childhood/adolescent breast cancer.[20]
- **Genetic risk:** Breast self-examination in the adolescent population is controversial but is recommended for girls who carry **the *BRCA1* or *BRCA2* gene** beginning at age 18 to 21 years.[15]
- **Immunocompromised patients:** Patients with diabetes, rheumatoid arthritis, or those using glucocorticoids may have an increased risk of breast infections.[9]

COMMONLY PRESCRIBED MEDICATIONS

TABLE 9.3 Commonly Prescribed Medications for Treatment of Breast Conditions in Adolescents

Medicine	Common Side Effects	Common Interactions
NSAIDs	▪ GI upset ▪ Recommend the patient take this with food.	▪ Avoid mixing with other NSAIDs
Hormonal contraceptives	▪ See related chapter	▪ See related chapter
Antibiotics ▪ Dosing and drug selection may vary. Check with provider regarding dosing/duration.	▪ Side effects will vary depending on the agent selected by the provider. ▪ Consult with a provider regarding any patient-reported side effects.	▪ Drug interactions will vary depending on the agent selected by the provider. ▪ Consult with a provider regarding medication interactions.

GI, gastrointestinal; NSAIDs, nonsteroidal anti-inflammatory drugs.

SUMMARY

Most breast symptoms in adolescents are benign.

▪ Breast asymmetry is common and is most pronounced during puberty. It can be monitored clinically and most often improves after puberty is complete.

▪ Breast discharge may be due to nipple stimulation, medications, pregnancy, an underlying breast mass, or idiopathic.

▪ Breast masses are typically benign, but malignancy should always be excluded, especially in high-risk populations.

▪ Breast tenderness is usually cyclic and can be managed expectantly with over-the-counter medications and certain comfort measures.

▪ A clinic evaluation should always be offered to the patient for assessment of her breast symptoms.

RELATED PROTOCOL

▪ Breast Ultrasounds are the preferred imaging in adolescents. Mammograms should not be performed.

References

1. Biro F, Greenspan L, Galvez M, et al. Onset of breast development in a longitudinal cohort. *Pediatrics.* 2013;132(6):1019. doi:10.1542/peds.2012–3773
2. Pitts S, Gordon C. The physiology of puberty. In: Emans SJ, Laufer MR, eds. *Goldstein's Pediatric & Adolescent Gynecology.* 6th ed. Philadelphia, PA: Lippincott Williams & Wilkins; 2012:100.

3. Committee on Practice Bulletins—Gynecology. Practice bulletin number 179: breast cancer risk assessment and screening in average-risk women. *Obstet Gynecol.* 2017;130(1):e1. doi:10.1097/AOG.0000000000002158

4. Greydanus D, Omar H, Pratt H. The adolescent female athlete: current concepts and conundrums. *Pediatr Clin North Am.* 2010;57(3):697–718. doi:10.1016/j.pcl.2010.02.005

5. Levinson W, Dunn P. Nonassociation of caffeine and fibrocystic breast disease. *Arch Intern Med.* 1986;146(9):1773. doi:10.1001/archinte.1986.00360210159022

6. Heyden S, Muhlbaier L. Prospective study of "fibrocystic breast disease" and caffeine consumption. *Surgery.* 1984;96(3):479.

7. Greydanus DE, Matytsina L, Gains M. Breast disorders in children and adolescents. *Prim Care.* 2006;33(2):455. doi:10.1016/j.pop.2006.02.002

8. Smith R, Pruthi S, Fitzpatrick L. Evaluation and management of breast pain. *Mayo Clin Proc.* 2004;79(3):353. doi:10.4065/79.3.353

9. Molitch M. Drugs and prolactin. *Pituitary.* 2008;11(2):209. doi:10.1007/s11102-008-0106-6

10. Baren JM. Breast lesions. In: Fleisher Ludwig S, Henretig FM, eds. *Textbook of Pediatric Emergency Medicine.* 5th ed. Philadelphia, PA: Lippincott Williams and Wilkins; 2006:193.

11. DiVasta AD, Weldon, C, Labow, BI. The brest: examination and lesions. In Emans SJ, Laufer MR, Goldstein, eds. *Pediatr and adolesc gynecol.* 6th ed. Philadelphia, PA: Lippincott Williams and Wilson. 2012: 412.

12. Simmons PS, Jayasinghe YL, Wold LE, Melton LJ III. Breast carcinoma in young women. *Obstet Gynecol.* 2011;118(3):529-536. doi:10.1097/AOG.0b013e31822a69db

13. Eidlitz-Markus T, Mukamel M, Haimi-Cohen Y, Amir J, Zehari A. Breast asymmetry during adolescence: physiologic and non-physiologic causes. *Isr Med Assoc J.* 2010;12(4):203-206.

14. De Silva NK, Brandt ML. Disorders of the breast in children and adolescents, part 1: disorders of growth and infections of the breast. *J Pediatr Adolesc Gynecol.* 2006;19(5):345. doi:10.1016/j.jpag.2006.06.006

15. Templeman C, Hertweck S. Breast disorders in the pediatric and adolescent patient. *Obstet Gynecol Clin North Am.* 2000;27(1):19. doi:10.1016/S0889-8545(00)80004-2

16. Faden H. Mastitis in children from birth to 17 years. *Pediatr Infect Dis J.* 2005;24(12):1113. doi:10.1097/01.inf.0000190031.59905.9f

17. DiVasta AD, Weldon C, Labow BI. The breast: examination and lesions. In: Emans SJ, Laufer MR, eds. *Goldstein's Pediatric & Adolescent Gynecology.* 6th ed. Philadelphia, PA: Lippincott Williams & Wilkins; 2012:405

18. Hodgson D, van Leeuwen F, Ng A, et al. Breast cancer after childhood, adolescent, and young adult cancer: it's not just about chest radiation. https://meetinglibrary.asco.org/record/138307/edbook#fulltext. Accessed June 27, 2019.

19. Schaapveld M, Aleman BM, van Eggermond AM, et al. Second cancer risk up to 40 years after treatment for Hodgkin's lymphoma. *N Engl J Med.* 2015;373:2499–2511. doi:10.1056/NEJMoa1505949

20. De Silva NK, Brandt ML. Disorders of the breast in children and adolescents, part 2: breast masses. *Pediatr Adolesc Gynecol.* 2006;19(6):415. doi:10.1016/j.jpag.2006.09.002

10

DYSMENORRHEA (MENSTRUAL CRAMPS)

Jeanette Higgins and Jane Geyer

INTRODUCTION

Dysmenorrhea, or pain during the menstrual period, is a common menstrual symptom among adolescent girls and young women. Dysmenorrhea is typically described as a crampy, suprapubic pain that begins before or during the menstrual period, although timing will vary between patients. Dysmenorrhea occurs in 20% to 90% of adolescent women.[1] Patients may report various degrees of perceived pain, and about 15% describe their pain as severe.[2] One third to one half of these women report moderate or severe symptoms. Dysmenorrhea can also be associated with nausea, vomiting, diarrhea, headaches, dizziness, back pain, and leg pain.[3] Treatment for primary dysmenorrhea should begin when medical care is sought.

CLINICAL PEARL BOX 1

Primary dysmenorrhea occurs after the establishment of ovulatory cycles. Ovulatory cycles generally occur 6 to 12 months after menarche.[3] Ovulatory cycles are believed to be associated with painful uterine contractions triggered by progesterone withdrawal at the beginning of the menses. These contractions result in uterine ischemia, causing pain that is derived from prostaglandins. These contractions vary in the length of time they last. Leukotrienes are also thought to have a role in dysmenorrhea as they are an inflammatory stimulant.

Secondary dysmenorrhea is defined as pain during the menstrual cycle due to pelvic pathology or a recognized medical condition. This may include but is not limited to infection, ovarian cysts, endometriosis, Mullerian anomalies, and obstructive reproductive tract anomalies.

COMMON PATIENT CONCERNS

- Menstrual pain
- Menstrual pain not improving with therapy

- Vomiting during menses
- Intermenstrual cramps
- Cyclic cramping in absence of menstruation

(O) KEY QUESTIONS TO ASK

- What age did menarche occur?
- How often does the patient have a menstrual period? How many days does the period last? How many pads or tampons does the patient use per day?
- Does the patient usually experience cramps with menses? If so, when did this start?
- When does the patient usually notice the onset of menstrual cramps (e.g., day before menses, first day of menses, etc.)?
- What would the patient rate the pain on a scale of 1 to 10? Has the patient been missing school or extracurricular activities because of her pain?
- Is the pain associated with any other symptoms such as nausea/vomiting, diarrhea, etc.?
- Which medications has the patient tried? Please include medication name, dose, frequency of dosing, and the patient's response to the medication.
- Is the patient sexually active?
- Does the patient experience cyclic pain intermenstrual? Or pain when not on her period?

TABLE 10.1 Patient Assessment for Dysmenorrhea

Acute Symptoms	Intervention/Delegation	Commonly Prescribed Medications
New onset or worsening of menstrual pain	Dysmenorrhea can occur and/or worsen when cycles become more ovulatory. The nurse should assess which over-the-counter medications the patient has tried taking and assess for adequate dosing. If the patient has not yet tried anything to help alleviate pain, the nurse can recommend a heating pad or OTC NSAIDs.[4,5] If the patient is not able improve their discomfort, they need to be evaluated in clinic.	NSAIDs Acetaminophen Heating pads

(continued)

TABLE 10.1 Patient Assessment for Dysmenorrhea (*continued*)

Acute Symptoms	Intervention/Delegation	Commonly Prescribed Medications
	For any severe pain not relieved with OTC medication, the patient should be referred to the ED. Encourage patient to keep a menstrual diary and pain diary to bring to the appointment.	
Vomiting with menses	Nausea/vomiting can occur in patients with dysmenorrhea.[3] The treatment for this is typically treating the dysmenorrhea. The nurse should assess which OTC medications the patient has tried taking and assess for adequate dosing. Encourage patient to keep a menstrual diary and pain diary to bring to the appointment	NSAIDs Acetaminophen

NSAIDs, nonsteroidal anti-inflammatory drug; OTC, over-the-counter.

TABLE 10.2 Chronic Symptoms of Dysmenorrhea

Chronic Symptoms	Nursing Counseling/Intervention	Commonly Prescribed Medications
Menstrual cramps	Heating pads, or heat therapy, have been shown to be effective at improving dysmenorrhea.[4,5] The nurse should suggest applying a topical heating pad if this is available to the patient. The nurse should assess which OTC medications the patient has tried taking and assess for adequate dosing. Oftentimes, inappropriate dosage or inappropriate scheduling of taking the medication can occur. The patient should make an office visit to discuss evaluation/treatment plan. Recommend the patient keep a menstrual calendar/pain journal to bring to the office visit. They could write this on a paper calendar or download an app to their phone.	NSAIDs Hormonal contraceptive options

(*continued*)

TABLE 10.2 Chronic Symptoms of Dysmenorrhea (*continued*)

Chronic Symptoms	Nursing Counseling/Intervention	Commonly Prescribed Medications
Intermenstrual cramps	This is usually cyclic, occurs mid-menstrual cycle, and is usually unilateral. Heating pads, or heat therapy has been shown to be effective at improving dysmenorrhea.[4,5] The nurse should suggest applying a topical heating pad, if this is available to the patient. The nurse should suggest exercising, as it has been shown to potentially helping to decrease pain severity; however, further research is needed.[6] The nurse should assess which OTC the patient has tried taking, and assess for adequate dosing. Recommend the patient keep a menstrual calendar/pain journal to bring to the upcoming office visit.	NSAIDs Hormonal contraceptive options
Vomiting with menses	Nausea/vomiting can occur in patients with dysmenorrhea. Treatment of dysmenorrhea typically improves N/V with menses, but if patient has not noticed an improvement after using NSAIDs + hormonal therapy for 3 months, please recommend patient make a follow-up visit.	NSAIDs OCPs
Cyclic cramping without menstruation	This is most likely secondary dysmenorrhea and clinical evaluation is recommended. The nurse can recommend the same comfort measures as with cramping with menstruation. Encourage the patient to keep a menstrual calendar and pain diary to bring to the upcoming office visit.	NSAIDs

NSAIDs, nonsteroidal anti-inflammatory drugs; N/V, nausea/vomiting; OTC, over the counter.

CLINICAL PEARL BOX 2

■ Patients who fail to respond to treatment with nonsteroidal anti-inflammatory drugs (NSAIDs) and hormonal therapy after three or more menstrual cycles should be evaluated for underlying causes of secondary dysmenorrhea.

➡ RED FLAGS

Pelvic pain: If someone is having lower abdominal or pelvic pain (suspicious for gynecologic origin) and not on their period, they should be referred to an urgent appointment in the office, their primary care physician (PCP), or urgent care/ED.

Heavy bleeding: If the patient is currently bleeding and is soaking one pad or one tampon per hour, and/or exhibiting signs/symptoms of anemia, refer the patient to the ED.

Nongynecological related pain: If the patient is experiencing a fever and/or vomiting, refer the patient to a PCP for evaluation.

TABLE 10.3 Commonly Prescribed Medicines for Treatment of Dysmenorrhea

Medication	Common Side Effects*
First line for dysmenorrhea: NSAIDs NSAIDs disrupt the production of prostaglandins, therefore should be the first line of treatment for the treatment of primary dysmenorrhea. Some adolescents respond better to Ibuprofen, others respond better to naproxen. The dose will depend on the weight and age of the adolescent.	Check for correct dosing and correct scheduling of medication. May cause GI upset; try taking with food and increase water.
Second line for dysmenorrhea: hormonal medications: Hormonal methods include oral contraceptive pills, patch, ring, injection, intrauterine devices, arm implant, or other oral or IM progesterone options. Extended cycling regimens are sometimes preferred.[7] Hormonal contraceptive options may be considered as first line in adolescent patients that are sexually active.[8]	See related hormonal therapy chapter(s) for side effects and management.

GI, gastrointestinal; IM, intramuscular; NSAIDs, nonsteroidal anti-inflammatory drugs.

*Consult with a provider regarding any patient-reported side effects

SUMMARY

- Primary dysmenorrhea is common in adolescent girls. It usually occurs once the cycles become ovulatory, which is about 6 to 12 months after menarche.
- Secondary dysmenorrhea is pain during the menstrual cycle due to pelvic pathology or a recognized medical condition.

■ It is important to try to identify whether it is primary dysmenorrhea or secondary dysmenorrhea. A patient with secondary dysmenorrhea may warrant sooner clinical evaluation.

■ The most common treatment options for dysmenorrhea include nonsteroidal anti-inflammatory drugs (NSAIDs) and hormonal therapy.

■ Most adolescents will report trying NSAIDs with little success, so always inquire about dosage typically used and timing, as most will report a suboptimal approach of NSAID therapy.

■ Further investigation is usually recommended in patients failing to respond to treatment after three or more menstrual cycles.

RELATED PROTOCOLS

■ Chapters 2, 3, 5, and 6: Hormonal Contraceptive
■ Chapter 13: Acute Pelvic Pain
■ Chapter 14: Chronic Pelvic Pain
■ Menstrual calendars

References

1. Emans SJ, Laufer, MR. Gynecologic pain: dysmenorrhea, acute and chronic pelvic pain, endometriosis, and premenstrual syndrome. In: *Pediatric & Adolescent Gynecology*. 6th ed. Philadelphia, PA: Lippincott Williams & Wilkins; 2012:238–241.
2. Sultan C, Gaspari L, Paris F. Adolescent dysmenorrhea. *Endocr Dev*. 2012;25(22): 171–180. doi:10.1159/000331775
3. ACOG Committee Opinion. Dysmenorrhea and endometriosis in the adolescent. *Obstet Gynecol*. 2018;132:e249–e258. doi:10.1097/AOG.0000000000002978
4. Akin M, Price W, Rodriguez G Jr, Erasala G, Hurley G, Smith RP. Continuous, low-level, topical heat wrap therapy as compared to acetaminophen for primary dysmenorrhea. *J Reprod Med*. 2004;49(9):739. doi:10.1016/s0029-7844(00)01163-7.
5. Akin MD, Weingand KW, Hengehold DA, Goodale MB, Hinkle RT, Smith RP. Continuous low-level topical heat in the treatment of dysmenorrhea. *Obstet Gynecol*. 2001;97(3):343. doi:10.1097/00006250-200103000-00004
6. Matthewman G, Lee A, Kaur JG, Daley AJ. Physical activity for primary dysmenorrhea: a systematic review and meta-analysis of randomized controlled trials. *Am J Obstet Gynecol*. 2018;219(3):255.e1. doi:10.1016/j.ajog.2018.04.001
7. Machado RB, de Melo NR, Maia H Jr. Bleeding patterns and menstrual-related symptoms with the continuous use of a contraceptive combination of ethinylestradiol and drospirenone: a randomized study. *Contraception*. 2010;81(3):215. doi:10.1016/j.contraception.2009.10.010
8. ACOG Committee Opinion No. 760 summary: dysmenorrhea and endometriosis in the adolescent. *Obstet Gynecol*. 2018;132(6):1517. doi:10.1097/AOG.0000000000002981

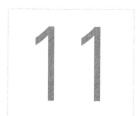

MAYER-ROKITANSKY-KUSTER-HAUSER SYNDROME

Kara Bendle and Deborah Morse

INTRODUCTION

Mayer-Rokitansky-Kuster-Hauser (MRKH) syndrome occurs in approximately one in 4,500 live female births.[1-3] It is characterized by the absence of a well-developed functioning uterus, a short or absent vagina, a female karyotype, with normal secondary sexual characteristics and ovarian function.[4] It results from the failure of the Mullerian ducts to fully mature in utero, resulting in a small or absent vagina and/or uterus.[1-3] It is important to note that the ovaries come from a different embryologic source, therefore their presence and function is almost always uncompromised.[3] The underlying cause of MRKH is unknown, although a combination of both genetic and environmental factors is suspected.[1-3]

MRKH is typically diagnosed when a young woman presents with primary amenorrhea, or menarche has failed to occur in the setting of appropriate pubertal development.[3,4] Young women may also present with a complaint of cyclic abdominal/pelvic pain if the uterine remnant has endometrium present. Imaging or laparoscopy can identify the presence of underdeveloped structures with active endometrium.

CLINICAL PEARL BOX

Mayer-Rokitansky-Kuster-Hauser (MRKH) can be associated with kidney, skeletal, hearing, and heart anomalies; it is important to assess and evaluate for these possible associated conditions.[1-3]

Menstrual suppression interventions such as oral contraceptive pills or a gonadotropin-releasing hormone (GnRH) agonist can be utilized to prevent the accumulation of obstructed menstruation while surgical planning is underway on those patients with a functional uterine remnant. Oral contraceptives can be utilized to combat cyclic pelvic pain caused by ovulation and residual endometriosis.[3]

This diagnosis can be devastating for an adolescent and her family; therefore, it is best to wait to initiate treatment until the time that the patient is physically and emotionally mature. Education should be patient-led, individualized, and offered when she herself chooses to move forward with therapy, usually in adolescence or early adulthood.[3,5] Nonsurgical progressive perineal dilation is the first-line treatment recommended to create a functional vaginal space. It is a patient-driven technique that is easy to perform, cost-effective, and safe.[3,6] Successful neovaginal creation by dilation eliminates the need for major surgery in most patients. Patient refusal or inability to perform vaginal dilations should not dictate the decision to pursue surgical vaginoplasty. Most surgical interventions require pre- and postoperative dilation to establish comfort with dilations prior to the procedure and to maintain vaginal patency after.[3,4] If surgical intervention becomes necessary, referral to a center with surgical expertise is recommended.[3]

Young women with MRKH who become sexually active should be counseled about the risk of sexually transmitted infections. Condom use should be encouraged. Human papillomavirus (HPV) vaccination is recommended to decrease the risk of developing vulvar/vaginal lesions and genital warts.[3]

Processing the initial diagnosis and adhering to vaginal dilations can heighten a young woman's concerns about her sexuality and fertility. It is important for the nurse to provide reliable resources and reassurance, but additional support from interdisciplinary team members such as behavioral medicine, social work, and pelvic floor physical therapy may be important referrals to integrate into the patient's care. Utilizing social services to connect the patient and family to others with an MRKH or similar diagnosis as a peer-to-peer opportunity is often beneficial. Social media support groups and chat rooms may provide other opportunities for teens to receive support and learn more about their health condition.[6]

COMMON PATIENT CONCERNS

- ▪ Anxiety/depression
- ▪ Bleeding/discharge while dilating
- ▪ Pain while dilating
- ▪ Urinary tract symptoms while dilating
- ▪ Mold fails to stay in place postop
- ▪ Postoperative concerns (further discussed in Postoperative chapter, Chapter 17)
- ▪ Pain/discomfort prior to any intervention
- ▪ Vaginal concerns with sexual activity/intercourse

⊙ KEY QUESTIONS TO ASK

Upon diagnosis

- Has the patient ever had any vaginal bleeding?
- Does the patient have any complaints of cyclic (approximately once a month at/around the same time of the month) or chronic abdominal or pelvic pain?
- When did the patient start breast development?
- When did the patient start to have axillary (armpit) hair?
- Does the patient have hearing loss or difficulty hearing?
- Has the patient ever been told that she has a heart problem?
- Does the patient have any bone/skeletal issues, such as scoliosis?

When dilating

- Does the patient have bleeding?
- Does the patient have pain?
- Does the patient have urinary symptoms such as frequency, urgency, pain, or incontinence?
- Does the patient have vaginal discharge?
- Has the patient attempted sexual intercourse?
- Has the patient been successful in identifying a private space in which to dilate?
- Has the patient's privacy been respected by other family members?
- Does the patient's schedule allow the time for dilation?

After surgical creation of a neovagina

- Does the patient have pain? Has the patient taken any prescribed or over-the-counter medications? When was the last dose?
- Does the patient have bleeding? How heavy is it? How long has it been going on?
- When was the patient's last bowel movement?
- Has the patient had difficulty wearing the vaginal mold or dilating as recommended?

PATIENT ASSESSMENT

Upon diagnosis

- Assess knowledge deficit
- Assess degree of anxiety/depression

When dilating

- Assess presence/severity of bleeding
- Assess presence/level of pain

- Assess presence/degree of urinary tract symptoms
- Assess patient's perception of the dilating experience
- If the patient has become sexually active, assess for difficulty with sexual activity
- If the patient has become sexually active, assess for use of condoms
- If the patient has become sexually active, assess for vaginal discharge

After surgical creation of a neovagina

- After hospital discharge, ensure that the patient has a postoperative appointment scheduled.
- Assess resumption of vaginal dilations after postoperative appointment (approximately 3 to 4 weeks after procedure)
- Assess for presence of and severity of bleeding
- Assess for presence of and degree of pain
- Assess patient's perception of the dilating experience
- If the patient has become sexually active, assess for difficulty with sexual activity
- If the patient has become sexually active, assess for the use of condoms
- If the patient has become sexually active, assess for vaginal discharge

TABLE 11.1 Symptoms of Mayer-Rokitansky-Kuster-Hauser Syndrome

Acute Symptoms	Intervention/Delegation	Commonly Prescribed Medicine
Bleeding/discharge while dilating	Schedule an urgent office visit if bleeding/discharge is severe. If the bleeding/discharge is not severe or if it resolves after the dilating session, recommend increased use of lubrication when dilating.[3,7]	Lubricant (K-Y® jelly, coconut oil)[7]
Pain while dilating	Schedule an urgent office visit if pain is severe. If pain is not severe or persistent after discontinuing the dilating session, recommend use of lidocaine jelly as lubricant or increased use of a lubricant when dilating.[3,7]	Lubricant (K-Y® jelly, coconut oil)[7] Lidocaine jelly[6]
Urinary tract symptoms while dilating	Schedule an urgent office visit if urinary tract symptoms are persistent or if persistent discharge is present.[3,7]	Antibiotics as indicated per provider

(continued)

TABLE 11.1 Symptoms of Mayer-Rokitansky-Kuster-Hauser Syndrome (*continued*)

Acute Symptoms	Intervention/Delegation	Commonly Prescribed Medicine
Mold fails to stay in place postop	Recommend changing undergarment type (boyshorts, thong) or size. Schedule an office visit for persistent difficulty.	
Postop bleeding	If the bleeding is severe, schedule an urgent office visit or refer the patient to the ED per office protocol. **See Chapter 17: Postoperative Concerns**	
Postop pain	Assess the patient's adherence to the prescribed medication regimen. Recommend adherence to prescribed medication regimen. If the pain is severe, schedule an urgent office visit or refer the patient to the ED per office protocol. **See Chapter 17: Postoperative Concerns**	Pain medications as indicated per provider
Postop urinary tract symptoms	Recommend an office visit to test for urinary tract infections. **See Chapter 17: Postoperative Concerns**	Antibiotics as indicated per provider
Postop constipation	Assess the duration and frequency of postop meds. Recommend the patient wean off narcotic prescription medications as tolerated. Increase high fiber foods in the diet. Increase activity as tolerated. **See Chapter 17: Postoperative Concerns**	Stool softeners Laxatives

TABLE 11.2 ED Considerations for Mayer-Rokitansky-Kuster-Hauser Syndrome

Chronic Symptoms/ Concerns	Intervention/Delegation	Commonly Prescribed Medicine
Anxiety/depression	Refer the patient to counseling and/ or peer support group. Reassure the patient that these feelings are common for young women receiving this diagnosis. Discuss strategies to share the diagnosis with family, friends, and partners.[3]	
Pain/discomfort prior to any intervention	Schedule an office visit. Check with a provider to see if imaging prior to the appointment is appropriate.	Oral contraceptive pills GnRH agonist
Mild/intermittent bleeding while dilating	Suggest increased use of lubricant (use water-soluble lubricant without additives).[3] Switch to a wider or softer dilator.[3] Suggest a temporary, short suspension of dilating.[3]	Lubricant (K-Y® jelly, coconut oil)[7]
Mild pain/discomfort while dilating	Suggest increased use of lubricant (use water-soluble lubricant without additives).[3] Switch to a wider or softer dilator.[3]	Lubricant (K-Y® jelly, coconut oil)[7]
Displeasure/general difficulty with dilating	Explore areas causing difficulty, i.e., lack of motivation, lack of supportive peer or family relationships, sociocultural issues, unresolved feelings of grief and/ or loss, knowledge deficit of diagnosis and/or dilating procedure, lack of private setting for dilating, transportation issues for office follow up.[3] Brainstorm strategies to overcome challenges/provide encouragement.[3] Suggest counseling/peer support group.[3] Discuss relaxation techniques (playing favorite background music, taking a warm bath, etc.).[7] Refer the patient to an experienced pelvic floor therapist.[3,6]	

(continued)

TABLE 11.2 ED Considerations for Mayer-Rokitansky-Kuster-Hauser Syndrome (*continued*)

Chronic Symptoms/Concerns	Intervention/Delegation	Commonly Prescribed Medicine
Vulvar, vaginal irritation with/after intercourse	Recommend condom use.[3] Suggest increased use of a lubricant[3]	Lubricant (K-Y® jelly, coconut oil)[7]
Vulvar, vaginal discharge with/after intercourse	Schedule an office visit to test for an infection.[3]	
Difficulty with sexual activity after discontinuation of dilating	Reassure the patient that intermittent but temporary pauses in dilating are not detrimental long term.[3] Encourage the patient to resume dilating with the largest comfortable dilator and increase dilator size as tolerated.[3] Reassure the patient that the frequency of dilating can decrease as the regularity of sexual intercourse increases.[3] Suggest increased use of lubricant (use water-soluble lubricant without additives).[3]	Lubricant (K-Y® jelly, coconut oil)[3,7]
	Reassure the patient that these feelings are common for young women receiving this diagnosis and that the genetic profile, internal reproductive organs other than the uterus and vagina, along with hormone production is female.[2,3]	

GnRH, gonadotropin-releasing hormone.

RED FLAGS

■ **Chronic cyclic abdominal/pelvic pain** could be an indication of active endometrium in rudimentary Mullerian structures, ovulation, an obstructed outflow tract, or endometriosis.[3] If the patient is stable, the nurse should assist in scheduling an office visit for evaluation.

■ **Acute, persistent pain** could be an indication of an obstructed outflow tract.[3] If the pain is severe, the patient should be evaluated in the ED.

■ **Acute, persistent bleeding** could be an indication of a vaginal abrasion or laceration.[3] If the bleeding is heavy, the patient should be instructed to seek evaluation at an ED.

■ **Urinary frequency, urgency, or pain upon urination** could be an indication of a urinary tract infection or urethral irritation/injury.[3] The patient should be evaluated in clinic.

■ **Persistent vaginal discharge** could be an indication of infection.[3] The patient should be evaluated in clinic.

TABLE 11.3 Commonly Prescribed Medicines for Treatment of Mayer-Rokitansky-Kuster-Hauser Syndrome

Medicine	Common Side Effects	Common Interactions
NSAIDs	Gastrointestinal distress, bleeding[8]	Not recommended for use in patients with certain renal conditions[8] Can decrease the therapeutic effect of certain diuretics and antihypertensives[8] Use with Warfarin can increase INR[8]
Acetaminophen		Use with Warfarin can increase INR[9] Avoid use with alcohol[9]
Laxative	Nausea, vomiting, abdominal cramps[10]	May cause laxative dependence and depletion of fluid and electrolytes[10]
Stool softener	Abdominal cramping, diarrhea[11]	No serious adverse effects[11]
Hormonal contraceptives	See Chapters 2, 3, 5, and 6 on hormonal contraception	See Chapters 2, 3, 5, and 6 on hormonal contraception
GnRH agonist (Lupron Depot®)	Generalized pain, injection site reaction, hot flashes/sweats, GI disorders, joint disorders[12]	No pharmacokinetic-based drug-drug interaction studies have been conducted[12]

GI, gastrointestinal; GnRH, gonadotropin-releasing hormone; INR, international normalized ratio; NSAIDs, nonsteroidal anti-inflammatory drugs.

MANAGING SIDE EFFECTS

It is important to instruct patients to track any signs or symptoms and to adhere to medication regimens as prescribed. Patients and caregivers should be instructed that medication regimens can be altered and changed if adverse side effects occur.[13] The nurse should consult with a provider if the patient reports any side effects.

SUMMARY

■ With the proper support and encouragement, 90% to 96% of young women can successfully create an anatomically and functional neovagina with progressive perineal dilation.[3]

■ The role of the office/triage nurse is to alleviate questions or concerns and to empower healthcare maintenance.

■ Follow-up visits are critical to establishing a therapeutic relationship between the patient and healthcare providers. Clinic visits are also necessary to ensure dilator adherence and track progress of the dilation.[6]

▨ When a surgical intervention is necessary, the patient should be followed with a pediatric and adolescent gynecology surgeon with expertise, as a successful outcome is greater with the initial procedure than with follow-up procedures.[3]

RELATED PROTOCOLS

▨ Chapter 17: Postoperative Concerns
▨ Chapter 13: Acute Pelvic Pain
▨ Chapter 14: Chronic Pelvic Pain

References

1. Fontana L, Gentilin B, Fedele L, Gervasini C, Miozzo M. Genetics of Mayer-Rokitansky-Küster-Hauser (MRKH) syndrome. *Clin Genet.* 2016;91(2):233–246. doi:10.1111/cge.12883
2. National Institutes of Health. Mayer-Rokitansky-Kuster-Hauser syndrome. https://ghr.nlm.nih.gov/condition/mayer-rokitansky-kuster-hauser-syndrome#statistics. Accessed February 6, 2018.
3. American College of Obstetricians and Gynecologists. ACOG committee opinion no. 728: Mullerian agenesis: diagnosis, management and treatment. *Obstet Gynecol.* 2018;131:e35-e42. doi:10.1097/AOG.0000000000002458
4. Yasmin E, Busby G. Mayer-Rokitansky-Kuster-Hauser syndrome. In: Creighton SM, Belen A, Breech L, Liao LM, eds. *Pediatric and Adolescent Gynecology: A Problem-Based Approach.* New York, NY: Cambridge University Press; 2018:99–108.
5. Nakhal RS, Creighton SM. Management of vaginal agenesis. *J Pediatr Adolesc Gynecol.* 2012;25:352-357. doi:10.1016/j.jpag.2011.06.003
6. Thomas P, Burke V, Jenks Micheli A. Education of the child and adolescent. In: Emans SJ, Laufer MR, Goldstein DP, eds. *Pediatric & Adolescent Gynecology.* 5th ed. Philadelphia, PA: Lippincott Williams & Wilkins; 2005:487–493.
7. North American Society for Pediatric and Adolescent Gynecology. NASPAG patient handout: Vaginal dilation. https://www.naspag.org/page/patienttools
8. *Motrin (Package Insert).* New York, NY: Pfizer, Inc.; 2007.
9. Food and Drug Administration. Organ-specific warnings; internal analgesic, antipyretic, and antirheumatic drug products for over-the counter human use; final monograph. *Fed Regist.* 2009;74(81):19385–19409.
10. Wilbur VF. Constipation, diarrhea, and irritable bowel syndrome. In: Archangel VP, Peterson AM, eds. *Pharmacotherapeutics for Advanced Practice: A Practical Approach.* 3rd ed. Philadelphia, PA: Lippincott Williams & Wilkins; 2013:424–453.
11. Adams M, Holland N, Urban C. Drugs for bowel disorders and other gastrointestinal conditions. In: Adams M, Holland N, Urban C, eds. *Pharmacology for Nurses: A Pathophysiologic Approach.* 5th ed. New York, NY: Pearson Education, Inc.; 2017:694–696.
12. *Lupron Depot (Package Insert).* Osaka, Japan: Takeda Pharmaceutical Company Limited; 2014.
13. Foy M, Peterson AM. Principles of pharmacology on pain management. In: Archangel VP, Peterson AM, eds. *Pharmacotherapeutics for Advanced Practice: A Practical Approach.* 3rd ed. Philadelphia, PA: Lippincott Williams & Wilkins; 2013:79–95.

12

OVARIAN CYSTS
Jeanette Higgins

INTRODUCTION

Ovarian cysts are often evaluated according to the patient's age. In the **antenatal period**, placental hormones and fetal hormones may stimulate the ovary.[1] After the baby is born, some cysts resolve while some cysts continue to enlarge.[1] Most of these cysts are detected with a prenatal ultrasound (US).[1] Treatment of these cysts have become less invasive with the aim of not harming the ovary.[1]

Ovarian cysts are not common in the **prepubertal female** because of low gonadotropin and sex hormone levels.[2] As puberty approaches, the incidence of ovarian cysts increases as a result of gonadotropin stimulation of the ovary.[3] Some functional cysts will activate hormones and result in a prepubertal child presenting with vaginal bleeding or premature breast development.[4] Nonfunctional ovarian cysts also occur in children and may not resolve without intervention.[4]

Functional cysts in the **pubertal females** are often a result of anovulation, with persistence of the remaining follicle and persistence of the corpus luteum.[5] Patients with symptomatic functional ovarian cysts may present with lower quadrant abdominal pain and/or menstrual irregularities. Functional ovarian cysts typically will resolve within 1 to 2 months.[5]

Ovarian and/or tubal torsion is rare, but is a surgical emergency.[6] Patients with severe abdominal pain with or without vomiting will likely need to be seen in the ED for evaluation of ovarian torsion and other underlying pathologies.[6]

CLINICAL PEARL BOX 1

Most physiologic ovarian cysts are benign and self-resolving without intervention. The majority of physiologic ovarian cysts resolve without treatment in 6 months.[2]

The risk of ovarian torsion increases when ovarian cysts/pelvic masses exceed 5 cm.[7]

CLINICAL PEARL BOX 2

Types of Ovarian Cysts*	Description/Counseling
Follicular/simple cysts	▪ Follicular/simple cysts are formed due to normal physiologic processes. ▪ These cysts usually resolve spontaneously. ▪ These cysts are usually discovered on ultrasound or other imaging. These patients can be seen in 4–6 weeks for follow up.
Complex cysts	▪ Complex cysts are those that contain blood or a solid substance. ▪ A ruptured vessel in the highly vascular corpus luteum may cause corpus luteal hemorrhagic cysts. This can cause acute severe pain and sometimes nausea due to acute distention of the capsule. ▪ These cysts usually resolve spontaneously. They can look complex on ultrasound and can be mistaken for a dermoid cyst. ▪ Most ovarian cysts are not cancerous. ▪ Patients with complex cysts need an appointment and repeat imaging.
Ovarian cysts in prepubertal patients	▪ Cysts in prepubertal children can occur. ▪ Prepubertal children with vaginal bleeding and a cyst need urgent evaluation or referral to the ED. ▪ Prepubertal children without vaginal bleeding also need evaluation, but it is not urgent.

*This chart is to be used for reference only. The provider will counsel and diagnose the patient depending on which type of cyst is present.

COMMON PATIENT CONCERNS

▪ Pain
▪ Irregular bleeding

⊙ KEY QUESTIONS TO ASK

Pain

▪ What would the patient rate the pain on a scale from 1 to 10 (1 being none)?

▪ When did the pain start?

▪ Where is the pain located?

▪ Can the patient describe the pain?

▪ Is this a new type of pain or a chronic type of pain?

▪ What interventions or medications has the patient tried to help alleviate the pain?

▪ Is the patient experiencing any associated nausea or vomiting with the pain?

Bleeding

▪ When did the bleeding start?

▪ How heavy is the bleeding? (see bleeding concerns chapter for further information)

▪ Is the patient experiencing any associated abdominal pain?

▪ Is the patient using any type of hormonal contraceptive option?

▪ Is the patient sexually active? If so, is there any chance of pregnancy or exposure to a sexually transmitted infection (STI)?

PATIENT ASSESSMENT

TABLE 12.1 Symptoms of Ovarian Cysts

Symptoms	Counseling/Nursing Intervention	Common Medications Prescribed
Pain	If the pain is severe, the patient should be referred to the ED. Pain that is not severe can be treated with over the counter medications, heating pads, and/or warm baths. The nurse should obtain any imaging completed for the provider to review.	NSAIDs Acetaminophen Heating pads
Nausea/vomiting	Nausea and vomiting are reported in 62%–67% of torsion cases.[7] These patients with nausea and vomiting should be referred to the ED for assessment.	

(continued)

TABLE 12.1 Symptoms of Ovarian Cysts (*continued*)

Symptoms	Counseling/Nursing Intervention	Common Medications Prescribed
Bleeding	This may be due to a multitude of underlying conditions.	
	Bleeding can occur with a germ-cell tumor due to estrogen production.[4]	
	A clinical evaluation is maybe indicated if this bleeding is not a regular menstrual period or menarche.	
	The nurse should obtain any imaging completed for the provider to review.	

NSAIDs, nonsteroidal anti-inflammatory drugs.

➡ RED FLAGS

Ovarian Torsion: All patients with torsion present with abdominal pain. The most common clinical symptom of torsion is sudden onset abdominal pain that is intermittent.[7] Nausea and vomiting are more commonly reported with torsion than with a cyst alone.[7] Clinical signs of torsion include abdominal tenderness.[7] These patients should be referred to the ED.

Malignancy: Patients with abdominal pain, increasing abdominal girth, nausea, and vomiting should be assessed for an ovarian tumor. These patients need to be seen urgently or referred to the ED. Patients with a palpable mass, bloating, and distention need to be seen urgently or referred to the ED for evaluation as this could represent an ovarian tumor.

Tubal pregnancy: Tubal pregnancy or ectopic pregnancy occurs in 2% of all first-trimester pregnancies.[5] Patients with abdominal pain, vaginal bleeding, and a missed period need to be referred to the ED. Other clinical presentations may include nausea and/or breast tenderness. The patient may not be aware she is pregnant.

TABLE 12.2 Commonly Prescribed Medicines for Treatment of Ovarian Cysts

Medicine	Common Side Effects*
Ibuprofen	Check for correct dosing and correct scheduling of medication.
	May cause GI upset; try taking with food and increase water.

(*continued*)

TABLE 12.2 Commonly Prescribed Medicines for Treatment of Ovarian Cysts (*continued*)

Medicine	Common Side Effects*
Naproxen	Check for correct dosing and correct scheduling of medication. May cause GI upset; try taking with food and increase water.
Hormonal medications	See chapter as related.

GI, gastrointestinal.

*Consult with a provider regarding any patient-reported side effects.

SUMMARY

▨ Age, pubertal status, and symptoms will help determine the possible origin of the cyst, and how soon the patient needs to be seen.

▨ Most patients with ovarian cysts have a favorable outcome without any intervention.

▨ Ovarian torsion should always be considered in patients with severe pain, with or without associated nausea/ vomiting.

▨ Malignancy may be rare, but should always be excluded in patients presenting with ovarian cysts.

RELATED PROTOCOLS

▨ Chapter 7: Birth Control: Intrauterine Devices

▨ Chapter 8: Bleeding Concerns

▨ Chapter 13: Acute Pelvic Pain

▨ Chapter 15: Polycystic Ovary Syndrome

References

1. Bagolan P, Giorlandino C, Nahom A, et al. The management of fetal ovarian cysts. *J Pediatr Surg*. 2002;37(1):25–30. doi:10.1053/jpsu.2002.29421

2. Schallert EK, Abbas PI, Mehollin-Ray AR, et al. Physiologic ovarian cysts versus other ovarian and adnexal pathologic changes in the preadolescent and adolescent population: US and surgical follow-up. *Radiology*. 2019;292(1):172–178. doi:10.1148/radiol.2019182563

3. Emeksiz HC, Derinoz O, Akkoyun EB, et al. Age-specific frequencies and characteristics of ovarian cysts in children and adolescents. *J Clin Res Pediatr Endocrinol*. 2017;9(1):58–62. doi:10.4274/jcrpe.3781

4. Aydin BK, Saka N, Bas, F, et al. Evaluation and treatment results of ovarian cysts in childhood and adolescence: a multicenter, retrospective study of 100 patients. *J Pediatr Adolesc Gynecol*. 2017;30(4):449–455. doi:10.1016/j.jpag.2017.01.011

5. Emans SJ, Laufer MR. Adnexal masses: ovarian cysts. In: *Pediatric & Adolescent Gynecology*. 6th ed. Philadelphia, PA: Lippincott Williams & Wilkins; 2012:384–388.

6. Hernon M, McKenna J, Busby G, et al. The histology and management of ovarian cysts found in children and adolescents presenting to a children's hospital from 1991 to 2007: a call for more paediatric gynaecologists. *BJOG*. 2010;117(2):181–184. doi:10.1111/j.1471-0528.2009.02433.x
7. ACOG Committee Opinion. *Adnexal torsion in adolescents. Am Coll Obstetric Gyn.* 2019;134:e56–63.

13

ACUTE PELVIC PAIN
Abigail Smith and Krista Childress

INTRODUCTION

It is estimated that adolescent females account for approximately eight million ED visits annually, with lower abdominal pain or genitourinary symptoms among the most common chief complaints.[1] Acute pelvic pain is defined as pain occurring for less than 3 months.[2] In an adolescent, acute pelvic warrants prompt evaluation and management given that several etiologies include conditions that may require urgent intervention.[3]

Acute pelvic pain can be caused by a wide array of diagnoses; therefore, it is important to evaluate all organ systems as a source for this pain. The differential diagnoses of acute pelvic pain include gynecologic, urologic, gastrointestinal, psychological, musculoskeletal, and infectious disease origins.[3]

Acute pelvic pain can cause anxiety for both patients and their guardians, so it is imperative that an accurate history is obtained in order to determine the origin or the pain. The role of the triage nurse is to help manage the patient's symptoms and answer questions regarding the patient's treatment. It is also the role of the triage nurse to determine if the symptoms warrant evaluation in the ED.

> ### CLINICAL PEARL BOX
> If acute pelvic pain is not managed at home with scheduled nonsteroidal anti-inflammatory drugs and/or the patient has associated fever, nausea, and/or vomiting, ED evaluation is warranted.

COMMON PATIENT CONCERNS

- Adnexal cysts
- Endometriosis
- Sexually transmitted infection
- Appendicitis
- Pregnancy

(O) KEY QUESTIONS TO ASK

- When did the pain begin?
- Was the patient doing any activity when the pain began?
- Where is the pain located and does it radiate anywhere?
- Is the pain above or below the umbilicus?
- In which quadrant is the pain located?
- How long has the pain been present?
- What is the pain rated on a scale from 1 to 10?
- Does any activity make it better or worse?
- What treatment option has the patient tried? Does anything help the pain? If patient is using nonsteroidal anti-inflammatory drugs (NSAIDs) or other pain medications, please note dose and frequency.
- Is the patient sexually active? If so, is there any chance of pregnancy? What method of contraception is currently being used by the patient?
- Is the patient experiencing abnormal vaginal discharge?
- When was the patient's last menstrual period?
- Are there any associated urinary symptoms such as dysuria, frequency, urgency?
- When was the patient's last bowel movement (BM)? How often does the patient have a BM? Does the patient have straining associated with BMs?
- Has there been any recent physical activity that could have strained a muscle? Any new sport, workout, outdoor work, new job?
- Has the patient had any recent surgeries or procedures?
- Is the patient under stress? Does the patient suffer from anxiety and/or depression? Is there a history of abuse or trauma?

PATIENT ASSESSMENT

TABLE 13.1 Symptoms of Acute Pelvic Pain

Symptoms	Intervention/Delegation	Commonly Prescribed Medicine
Pain associated with menses (dysmenorrhea)	If patient is currently menstruating and has not taken any pain medication, recommend use of scheduled NSAIDs such as ibuprofen or naproxen.[4] If use of NSAIDs is not sufficient or if dysmenorrhea is persistent, recommend evaluation in clinic for initiation of hormone therapy/contraception to treat symptoms.	NSAIDs Hormone therapy/contraception

(continued)

TABLE 13.1 Symptoms of Acute Pelvic Pain (*continued*)

Symptoms	Intervention/Delegation	Commonly Prescribed Medicine
Sudden onset of severe abdominal pain with associated nausea and/or vomiting	Common gynecologic etiologies: adnexal cyst, ruptured adnexal cyst, adnexal torsion. The most common clinical symptom of adnexal torsion is the sudden onset of abdominal pain with nausea and vomiting.[5] Appendicitis can present with similar symptoms, which also warrants evaluation in the ED as the patient may require surgical intervention.[2] If NSAIDs are ineffective at managing pain recommend evaluation in the ED.	Adnexal torsion is a surgical emergency warranting diagnostic laparoscopy for untwisting.[5]
Pelvic pain in sexually active patient	Adolescents are at a higher risk of PID because of high-risk sexual behaviors.[2] STIs such as *Chlamydia trachomatis* and *Neisseria gonorrhoeae* can be asymptomatic and can lead to PID.[4] If the patient is suspected to have PID, it is important they are evaluated promptly in clinic or in the ED. Ectopic pregnancy must also be considered in sexually active females reporting pelvic pain, especially if associated with abnormal uterine bleeding.[3] If concerned for ectopic pregnancy, patient needs immediate evaluation in ED or clinic.	Treatment of sexually transmitted infections and/or PID: Azithromycin Ceftriaxone Doxycycline Metronidazole Ectopic Pregnancy: Can be managed via medical or surgical modalities, which is determined based on patient status and other clinical factors.[2]
Pelvic pain associated with constipation	Constipation is one of the most common causes of abdominal pain and can occur in all age groups[7] Bowel movements should occur daily and be soft and easy to pass without straining. If patient is constipated, recommend increased fluid intake and use of a stool softener.[8]	Stool softeners

(*continued*)

TABLE 13.1 Symptoms of Acute Pelvic Pain (*continued*)

Symptoms	Intervention/Delegation	Commonly Prescribed Medicine
Pelvic pain associated with urinary symptoms	If patient is afebrile and experiencing pain with urination, recommend evaluation in clinic for possible urinary tract infection.[2,7] If patient is febrile and has associated urinary symptoms, recommend evaluation in the ED as this is concerning for pyelonephritis.[2,7]	

NSAIDs, nonsteroidal anti-inflammatory drugs; PID, pelvic inflammatory disease; STI, sexually transmitted infection.

➡ RED FLAGS

Any severe pain that is not managed with scheduled NSAIDs, especially with associated nausea and vomiting, should be seen in the ED.

Any time a fever is accompanying pain, an urgent evaluation should be considered, especially in patients who are sexually active.

Any sexually active patient with concern for pregnancy should be evaluated promptly.

⊙ SPECIAL POPULATION CONSIDERATIONS

Special needs: There are a number of patients with special needs who are unable to describe their symptoms and it is often the caregiver that voices concerns on behalf of the patient. It is important to listen to the caregivers and determine if the symptoms presented warrant an in-clinic or ED evaluation.

TABLE 13.2 Commonly Prescribed Medicines for Treatment of Acute Pelvic Pain

Medicine	Common Side Effects*
NSAIDs	▪ Check for correct dosing and scheduling of medication. ▪ May cause GI upset. Take with food and increase fluid intake.
Hormone therapy/ Contraception	▪ See Chapters 2–7.
Polyethylene glycol	▪ These are stool softeners and must be taken with fluids in order to work appropriately.

GI, gastrointestinal; NSAIDs, nonsteroidal anti-inflammatory drugs.

*Consult with a provider regarding any patient-reported side effects.

SUMMARY

▨ Pelvic pain is a common condition in the adolescent gynecology population.

▨ Acute pelvic pain is pain that has been occurring for ≤3 months.

▨ Certain etiologies of pelvic pain can require emergent intervention and it is important to determine if a patient needs immediate evaluation in the ED.

▨ If acute pelvic pain is not managed at home with scheduled NSAIDs and/ or has associated fever, nausea, and/or vomiting, the patient warrants evaluation in the ED.

RELATED PROTOCOLS

▨ Chapter 10: Dysmenorrhea (Menstrual Cramps)
▨ Chapter 14: Chronic Pelvic Pain
▨ Chapter 16: Positive Pregnancy Test
▨ Chapter 12: Ovarian Cysts

References

1. Goyal MK, Rowlett JD. *AM:STARs Acute Emergencies in Adolescents*. Vol. 26. 3rd ed. Itasca, IL: American Academy of Pediatrics; 2016.
2. Kruszka PS, Kruszka SJ. Evaluation of acute pelvic pain in women. *Am Fam Physician*. 2010;82(2):141–147.
3. Emans SJ, Laufer MR, Goldstein DP. *Pediatric and Adolescent Gynecology*. Philadelphia, PA: Wolters Kluwer Health; 2015.
4. Sanctis VD, Soliman A, Bernasconi S, et al. Primary dysmenorrhea in adolescents: prevalence, impact and recent knowledge. *Pediatr Endocrinol Rev*. 2015;13(2):512–520.
5. Adnexal torsion in adolescents. *Obstet Gynecol*. 2019;134(2):e56–e63. doi:10.1097/aog.0000000000003373
6. Oltmann SC, Fischer A, Barber R, Huang R, Hicks B, Garcia N. Cannot exclude torsion—a 15-year review. *J Pediatr Surg*. 2009;44(6):1212–1216. doi:10.1016/j.jpedsurg.2009.02.028
7. Reust CE, Williams A. Acute abdominal pain in children. *Am Fam Physician*. 2016;93(10):830–837.
8. Biggs WS, Dery WH. Evaluation and treatment of constipation in infants and children. *Am Fam Physician*. 2006;73:469–477.

14

CHRONIC PELVIC PAIN
Jane Geyer and Jeanette Higgins

INTRODUCTION

Pelvic pain constitutes nearly 3% to 5% of all primary care visits.[1] Pelvic pain can be acute or chronic. It is important to separate these issues to help determine the necessary treatment and the urgency of treatment. Chronic pelvic pain (CPP) is defined as pelvic pain occurring for least 6 months.[2,3]

All children and adolescents are susceptible to pelvic pain. CPP often requires a multi-disciplinary approach due to the vast amount of different etiologies. There are many underlying causes that may cause children or adolescents to experience chronic or persistent pelvic pain including gynecologic, urological, gastrointestinal, psychological, musculoskeletal, and/or infectious origins.

The workup for CPP is often similar to acute pelvic pain. The origin is not always easy to determine, leaving patients and their guardians frustrated. The role of the triage nurse is to help manage the patient's symptoms and answer questions they may have regarding treatment plans. It is also important to distinguish between new acute concerns that should be seen urgently from reoccurring symptoms that can be evaluated during a standard office visit.

Acute pelvic pain will be addressed separately.

COMMON PATIENT CONCERNS

- Worsening of dysmenorrhea
- Dysmenorrhea unresponsive to treatment options
- Suspected endometriosis
- Suspected ovarian cyst or lesions
- Pelvic pain associated with urinary concerns
- Pelvic pain associated with constipation

⊙ KEY QUESTIONS TO ASK

- When did the pain begin?
- Where is the pain located? Is the pain above or below the umbilicus? Which quadrant is the pain located?
- How often does the pain occur?
- What is the pain rated on a pain scale from 1 to 10?
- What treatment options has the patient tried (if patient using nonsteroidal anti-inflammatory drugs [NSAIDs] or pain meds, please note dose and frequency as well)? Does anything help the pain?
- Does anything make the pain worse?
- Is the patient sexually active? If so, is there any chance of pregnancy?
- Is the patient experiencing any vaginal discharge changes?
- Are there are any associated urinary symptoms such as dysuria, frequency, hesitancy?
- When was the patient's last bowel movement (BM)? How often does the patient have a BM? Does the patient have straining associated with BMs? Has the patient noticed blood in the stool?
- Has there been any recent physical activity that could have caused a strained muscle, such as sports, workouts, or outdoor work?
- Any recent surgeries or procedures?
- Is the patient under stress? Does the patient suffer from anxiety and/or depression? Is there a history of abuse or trauma?

PATIENT ASSESSMENT

TABLE 14.1 Symptoms and Patient Concerns for Chronic Pelvic Pain

Symptoms and Patient Concerns	Intervention/Delegation	Commonly Prescribed Medication
Worsening of dysmenorrhea and/or dysmenorrhea unresponsive to treatment options	■ Persistent dysmenorrhea not responding to NSAIDs and hormonal therapy after 3–6 months, often warrants a clinical evaluation.[4] ■ Up to 70% of adolescents with chronic pelvic/menstrual pain unresponsive to treatment are found to have endometriosis.[5] ■ The nurse should inquire about the dose and administration frequency of the pain-relieving medication that the patient has been taking. If the patient has	■ NSAIDs ■ Hormonal contraception ■ GnRH agonists (Depot Leuprolide Acetate) are used in patients with diagnosed endometriosis. ■ Add back therapy: Norethindrone acetate

(continued)

TABLE 14.1 Symptoms and Patient Concerns for Chronic Pelvic Pain (*continued*)

Symptoms and Patient Concerns	Intervention/Delegation	Commonly Prescribed Medication
	not been taking the dosage suggested by the provider and/or standard dosage, instruct the patient to do so. ▪ The nurse should inquire about which hormonal therapy option the patient is taking and ask appropriate questions to assess adherence (see related hormonal therapy in Chapter 3, if needed). Studies have not shown any OCPs to more effective than others in helping with dysmenorrhea. ▪ Using OCPs in a continuous manner vs cyclic manner may better help dysmenorrhea.[6]	
Suspected or diagnosed ovarian cysts	▪ Patients with a current ovarian cyst or history of ovarian cysts may complain of pain in the lower abdomen. ▪ Patients with functional cysts are typically managed expectantly. ▪ Provide reassurance that most cysts regress within two to three menstrual cycles.[7] ▪ If a patient is reporting a worsening or change in the abdominal pain since the most recent office visit, recommend the patient is reevaluated in clinic. ▪ The nurse should review torsion precautions with all patients with a known or suspected ovarian cyst. The most common clinical symptom of adnexal torsion is the sudden onset of abdominal pain with nausea and vomiting.[8] If torsion is suspected, patients should be sent to the nearest ED.	▪ NSAIDs ▪ Hormonal contraception

(*continued*)

TABLE 14.1 Symptoms and Patient Concerns for Chronic Pelvic Pain (*continued*)

Symptoms and Patient Concerns	Intervention/Delegation	Commonly Prescribed Medication
Pelvic pain associated with constipation	▣ The goal for most patients is to have a bowel movement every day without straining or difficulty. ▣ The patient should follow a diet that is conducive to regular bowel movements.[9] ▣ Although dietary changes have shown weak evidence for treatment of moderate to severe constipation, the nurse can encourage the patient to consume an adequate amount of clear fluids along with increasing fiber and fruits/vegetables in the diet.[10,11] ▣ An over-the-counter stool softener may be recommended in some patients. ▣ For patients that are following with a GI provider, ensure that the patient is following recommended bowel regimens and assess medication adherence. ▣ For patients that are not yet followed by a GI provider, recommend a follow up with the patient's primary care provider for a referral if deemed appropriate.	▣ Polyethylene glycol ▣ Docusate sodium
Pelvic pain associated with urinary concerns	▣ For patients with suspected or diagnosed urinary conditions such as painful bladder syndrome or kidney stones, the nurse can offer guidance of symptom relief strategies.[12] ▣ Encourage the patient to apply a heating pad to the lower abdomen. ▣ Avoid trigger foods/drinks which may include caffeine, spicy foods, citrus fruits/juices, artificial sweeteners. ▣ Encourage the patient to follow fluid intake instructions from their provider, as this is often individualized for each patient.	▣ NSAIDs ▣ Urinary analgesics

GI, gastroenterology; GnRH, gonadotropin releasing hormone; NSAIDs, nonsteroidal anti-inflammatory drugs.

➡ RED FLAGS

Patients experiencing severe pain that is not relieved with over-the-counter medication should always be evaluated in an ED.

Any time fever is accompanying pain, an ED evaluation should be considered, especially for those who are sexually active.

Females who not achieved menarche with pelvic pain need to be evaluated quickly. If your facility cannot accommodate this, they will need to be evaluated in the ED.

⊙ SPECIAL POPULATION CONSIDERATIONS

Special needs: Sometimes those with special needs are not able to describe their needs. Oftentimes, their caregivers are their voice, and we need to listen to the caregivers and their concerns.

History of pelvic inflammatory disease (PID): Up to 30% of patients with a history of PID will develop CPP.[13] Patients who are not responsive to standard pain regimens may require additional treatment options similar to practices used for neuropathic pain.[14]

Depression/Anxiety: Pelvic pain can occur with psychosocial alterations or in patients with anxiety/depression. Depression/anxiety can be both a cause and an effect of CPP.[15] Patients with a history of depression and/or anxiety need to be screened for suicidal ideations. If the patient discloses having a plan for suicide or self-harm, the patient should be sent to the nearest ED. Treatment of anxiety/depression with medication along with cognitive/behavior therapy may improve CPP.[15]

History of abuse or trauma: Patients with history of sexual abuse or trauma may have a higher risk of CPP.[16] Treatment of anxiety/depression with medication along with cognitive/behavior therapy may improve CPP.

TABLE 14.2 Commonly Prescribed Medications for Treatment of Chronic Pelvic Pain

Medicine	Common Side Effects
NSAIDs	May cause GI upset.
	Take with food and increase water.
Hormonal contraceptive options	See Chapters 2–7 as related.
GnRH agonist (Depot Leuprolide Acetate)	Hot flashes, sweating, decreased libido, breast tenderness, weight changes can occur.[17]
	Add back therapy with hormonal medications, such as norethindrone acetate, may help to decrease side effects.[18]

(continued)

TABLE 14.2 Commonly Prescribed Medications for Treatment of Chronic Pelvic Pain (*continued*)

Medicine	Common Side Effects
Polyethylene glycol Docusate sodium	Stool softeners should be taken with water in order for the medications to work properly.

GI, gastrointestinal; GnRH, gonadotropin releasing hormone; NSAIDs, nonsteroidal anti-inflammatory drugs.

SUMMARY

- CPP is a common condition in the adolescent GYN population and is defined as pelvic pain that has persisted for 6 months or more.
- It is often a multidisciplinary approach.
- Further evaluation of symptoms is often warranted sooner than 6 months, as young patients may be missing school and activities for their symptoms, therefore a prompt evaluation is encouraged.

RELATED PROTOCOLS

- Chapter 10: Dysmenorrhea (Menstrual Cramps)
- Chapter 13: Acute Pelvic Pain
- Chapter 16: Positive Pregnancy Test
- Chapter 12: Ovarian Cysts

References

1. Song AH, Advincula AP. Adolescent chronic pelvic pain. *J Pediatr Adolesc Gynecol.* 2005;18:371–377. doi:10.1016/j.jpag.2005.09.001
2. Royal College of Obstetricians and Gynaecologists. Green-top guideline No. 41: the initial management of chronic pelvic pain. May 2012. https://www.rcog.org.uk/globalassets/documents/guidelines/gtg_41.pdf. Accessed August 12, 2019.
3. American College of Obstetricians and Gynecologists. Frequently asked questions: gynecologic problems, FAQ099. August 2011. http://www.acog.org/Patients/FAQs/Chronic-Pelvic-Pain. Accessed December 19, 2016.
4. ACOG Committee Opinion. Number 310. Endometriosis in adolescents. *Obstet Gynecol.* 2005;105(4):921. doi:10.0.z1097/00006250-200504000-00058
5. Laufer MR, Goitein L, Bush M, Cramer DW, Emans SJ. Prevalence of endometriosis in adolescent girls with chronic pelvic pain not responding to conventional therapy. *J Pediatr Adolesc Gynecol.* 1997;10(4):199. doi:10.1016/S1083-3188(97)70085-8
6. Vercellini P, Frontino G, De Giorgi, et al. Continuous use of an oral contraceptive for endometriosis-associated recurrent dysmenorrhea that does not respond to a cyclic pill regimen. *Fertil Steril.* 2003;80(3):560. doi:10.1016/S0015-0282(03)00794-5
7. Kanizsai B, Orley J, Szigetvari I, et al. Ovarian cysts in children and adolescents: their occurrence, behavior, and management. *J Pediatr Adolesc Gynecol.* 1998;11:85. doi:10.1016/S1083-3188(98)70117-2

8. Adnexal torsion in adolescents: ACOG committee opinion no, 783. *Obstetr Gynecol.* 2019;134(2):e56–e63. doi:10.1097/aog.0000000000003373

9. Tabbers MM, DiLorenzo C, Berger M, et al. Evaluation and treatment of functional constipation in infants and children: evidence-based recommendations from ESPGHAN and NASPGHAN. *J Pediatr Gastroenterol Nutr.* 2014;58(2):258. doi:10.1097/MPG.0000000000000266

10. Young RJ, Beerman LE, Vanderhoof JA. Increasing oral fluids in chronic constipation in children. *Gastroenterol Nurs.* 1998;21(4):156. doi:10.1097/00001610-199807000-00002

11. Loening-Baucke V, Miele E, Staiano A. Fiber (glucomannan) is beneficial in the treatment of childhood constipation. *Pediatrics.* 2004;113(3 pt 1):e259. doi:10.1542/peds.113.3.e259

12. Hanno PM, Burks DA, Clemens JQ, et al. Guideline for the diagnosis and treatment of interstitial cystitis/bladder pain syndrome. *Interstitial Cystitis Guidelines Urol.* 2011;185(6):2162. doi:10.1016/j.juro.2011.03.064

13. Ness RB, Soper DE, Holley RL, et al. Effectiveness of inpatient and outpatient treatment strategies for women with pelvic inflammatory disease: results from the Pelvic Inflammatory Disease Evaluation and Clinical Health (PEACH) randomized trial. *Am J Obstet Gynecol.* 2002;186(5):929. doi:10.1067/mob.2002.121625

14. Gilron I, Baron R, Jensen T. Neuropathic pain: principles of diagnosis and treatment. *Mayo Clin Proc.* 2015;90(4):532. doi:10.1016/j.mayocp.2015.01.018

15. Powell J. The approach to chronic pelvic pain in the adolescent. *Obstetr Gynecol Clins.* 2014;41(3):343–355. doi:10.1016/j.ogc.2014.06.001

16. Walling MK, Reiter RC, O'Hara MW, et al. Abuse history and chronic pain in women: i. Prevalences of sexual abuse and physical abuse. *Obstet Gynecol.* 1994;84:193–199. doi:10.1016/0029-7844(94)p4403-b

17. Leuprolide. *Lexi-drugs. Lexicomp.* Riverwoods, IL: Wolters Kluwer Health, Inc. http://online.lexi.com. Accessed August 19, 2019.

18. Hornstein MD, Surrey ES, Weisberg GW, Casino LA. Leuprolide acetate depot and hormonal add-back in endometriosis: a 12-month study. Lupron Add-Back Study Group. *Obstet Gynecol.* 1998;91(1):16. doi:10.1016/S0029-7844(97)00620-0

15

POLYCYSTIC OVARY SYNDROME
Kara Bendle and Deborah Morse

INTRODUCTION

Polycystic ovary syndrome (PCOS) occurs in some females as the result of a hormone imbalance in which androgen levels are higher than normal. It embodies a broad range of presentations, but it is generally diagnosed in adolescents when menstrual irregularities are present with evidence of hyperandrogenism (clinical or laboratory).[1-3] PCOS can be difficult to diagnose in adolescents given some of the symptoms may mimic normal pubertal changes in females.

Elevated androgen levels can cause anovulation (failure of the monthly release of an egg from the ovary) and associated irregular or heavy periods. In addition, hyperandrogenism can cause acne, hirsutism (excessive body hair, especially on the face), and alopecia (hair loss). Patients with hyperandrogenism may also have acanthosis nigricans (a dark rash on the neck and/or axilla), and skin tags related to insulin excess.[2,3] The mainstay of treatment is achieving a normal body mass index (BMI), most times through diet and exercise. Hormonal contraception is often used to help control the symptoms of PCOS, with or without the addition of metformin in patients with associated insulin resistance.[2-4]

The prevalence of obesity in females diagnosed with PCOS in the United States is high, most likely due to a combination of both environmental and genetic factors, exacerbating insulin resistance and putting patients at greater risk for developing cardiovascular disease and type 2 diabetes.[2,3,5] Weight loss, exercise, and sometimes medications are recommended for overweight patients.[2,3]

Since regular ovulation and menstruation is affected, endometrial cancer and infertility are possible concerns of young women thinking about the future.[2,3] When patients do wish to become pregnant, keeping an accurate menstrual calendar, medications, and reproductive specialists can assist.[2,3]

While females diagnosed with PCOS are at a somewhat greater risk of developing endometrial cancer later in life, the American Cancer Society does not recommend special screening over and above the usual recommendations for regular well-woman care, being especially mindful of unexpected bleeding or spotting.[3,6]

COMMON PATIENT CONCERNS

- Acne
- Facial hair
- Neck rash
- Sadness/depression
- Menstrual irregularities
- Anxiety regarding fertility

KEY QUESTIONS TO ASK

- When was the patient's first period?
- How often does the patient have a period?
- When was the patient's last menstrual period (LMP)?
- How many days do the patient's periods last? How many pads/tampons does the patient change per day?
- Does the patient experience intermenstrual bleeding or spotting?
- Has the patient experienced weight gain and/or difficulty losing weight?
- Does the patient have acne? If so, where on the body does the patient notice this? Which over-the-counter options has the patient tried?
- Does the patient notice symptoms of hirsutism that bothers them?
- Is the patient sexually active?
- What over-the-counter and prescribed medications/supplements is the patient currently taking?

PATIENT ASSESSMENT

TABLE 15.1 Symptoms of Polycystic Ovary Syndrome

Chronic Symptoms/Concerns	Intervention/Delegation	Commonly Prescribed Medicine
Acanthosis nigricans	Schedule appointment with a provider to assess need for laboratory testing and/or hormonal medications.[2,3] Encourage compliance with prescribed medications.	Metformin

(continued)

TABLE 15.1 Symptoms of Polycystic Ovary Syndrome (*continued*)

Chronic Symptoms/ Concerns	Intervention/Delegation	Commonly Prescribed Medicine
	Emphasize that some medications may take a while before you see a reduction in symptoms. Reassure that medications can help control symptoms if caller has not yet been prescribed medications.	
Acne	Assess level of concern over symptoms.	Combined hormonal contraception[2,3]
	Schedule appointment with provider to assess need for hormonal or topical medications.[2,3]	Topical medications[2]
	Encourage compliance with prescribed medications.	
	Discuss mechanism of action of medications and advise compliance. Emphasize that some medications may take a while before you see a reduction in symptoms.	
	Reassure that medications can help control symptoms if caller has not yet been prescribed medications.	
Alopecia	Schedule appointment with provider to assess the need for laboratory testing and/or hormonal medications.[2,3]	Combined hormonal contraception[3]
	Encourage compliance with prescribed medications.	
Depression •	There appears to be a higher incidence of depression, anxiety, and panic disorders in women diagnosed with PCOS. [2,3]	
	Assess for depressive symptoms.	
	Reassure patient that these feelings are not unusual for young women diagnosed with PCOS.	
	Refer to appropriate mental health provider or peer support group.	
	Assess for suicidal ideations or thoughts/plans of self-harm or harming others. If the patient is experiencing any of these symptoms, the patient should be seen in the nearest ED.	

(*continued*)

TABLE 15.1 Symptoms of Polycystic Ovary Syndrome (*continued*)

Chronic Symptoms/ Concerns	Intervention/Delegation	Commonly Prescribed Medicine
Fertility concerns	Advise that the impact on fertility for everyone is uncertain, and when wishing to become pregnant, lifestyle changes and medications prescribed by a reproductive specialist can assist. Schedule an appointment with a provider to further discuss and answer additional questions the patient may have.	Ovulation stimulating medications
Hirsutism	Assess level of concern over symptoms. Schedule appointment with a provider to assess need for medications.[2-4] Ask if patient has been prescribed medications and is compliant with prescribed medication regime. Emphasize that some medications may take a while before you see a reduction in symptoms. Reassure that medications can help control symptoms if caller has not yet been prescribed medications.	Combined hormonal contraception[2-4] Spironolactone[4,7]
Insulin resistance or diabetes	Schedule appointment with provider to assess need for medications, specialist referrals, and/or updated laboratory testing.[2,3] Encourage exercise and weight loss.[2,3] Recommend the patient focus on a reduced calorie, low-carbohydrate, low-fat diet.[8] Encourage compliance with prescribed medications.	Metformin[2,3]
Menstrual irregularities	Recommend keeping menstrual calendar. Schedule appointment with provider to assess need for hormonal medications.[2,3] Encourage compliance with prescribed medications.	Hormonal contraception[2,3] Levonorgestrel IUD Cyclic progesterone[7]

(continued)

TABLE 15.1 Symptoms of Polycystic Ovary Syndrome (*continued*)

Chronic Symptoms/ Concerns	Intervention/Delegation	Commonly Prescribed Medicine
Obesity	Encourage weight loss strategies[2,3]	
	The nurse should be familiar with nutritional resources and/or nutritional/weight loss programs available to patients.	
	Schedule an appointment with a provider to discuss a weight loss plan and/or assess for the need for a referral to a specialist.	

IUD, intrauterine device; PCOS, polycystic ovary syndrome.

➡ RED FLAGS

- Unexpected vaginal bleeding/spotting-females diagnosed with PCOS have an increased relative risk for developing endometrial cancer later in life. Although routine screening with endometrial biopsy or ultrasound imaging is not recommended, bleeding outside of an expected menstrual period should be investigated.[3,6]

- Hypoglycemia (low blood sugar)—**acute** symptoms of dizziness, light-headedness, slow or irregular heartbeat, cold extremities, feeling tired or weak, feeling sleepy or drowsy, difficulty breathing, sudden stomach pains, nausea, or vomiting.[9]

- Lactic acidosis—**acute** symptoms of dizziness, lightheadedness, slow or irregular heartbeat, cold extremities, feeling tired or weak, feeling sleepy or drowsy, difficulty breathing, sudden stomach pains, nausea, or vomiting.[9]

TABLE 15.2 Special Population Considerations for Polycystic Ovary Syndrome

Condition	Special Intervention/ Delegation	Commonly Prescribed Medicine
Pregnancy—At risk for gestational diabetes, preterm delivery and preeclampsia.[2]	Referral to high-risk obstetrician **Spironolactone should not be used in pregnancy because of anti-androgenic effects on a male fetus.**[10]	

TABLE 15.3 Commonly Prescribed Medicines for Treatment of Polycystic Ovary Syndrome

Medicine	Common Side Effects*	Common Interactions
Metformin	GI distress: diarrhea, nausea/vomiting, flatulence, bloating, anorexia, indigestion, abdominal discomfort, headache, lack of energy, metallic taste in the mouth[9] Rare lactic acidosis[9]	Sulfonylurea—mild synergistic effect[9] Cimetidine—simultaneous use increases risk of hypoglycemia.[9] Glucocorticoids or alcohol—simultaneous use increases risk of lactic acidosis.[9] **Intravenous radiology contrast—receiving while taking metformin may result in acute decreased renal function and/or lactic acidosis.[9]**
Spironolactone	Hyperkalemia[10] Hypotension/decreased renal function[10] Electrolyte and metabolic abnormalities[10] Impaired neurologic function in patients with liver disorders[10] Anti-androgenic effects on a male fetus[4,10]	Potassium or drugs increasing serum potassium—concomitant use can lead to hyperkalemia.[10] Hormonal contraception containing drospirenone—should be used with caution in conjunction with spironolactone to avoid increased mineralocorticoid effects.[4] Lithium—concomitant use can lead to lithium toxicity.[10] NSAIDs—concomitant use can reduce the antihypertensive and antidiuretic effects of spirololactone.[10] Digoxin-can interfere with radioimmunologic assays of digoxin exposure.[10] Cholestyramine—concomitant use can lead to hyperkalemic metabolic acidosis.[10] Acetylsalicylic Acid—concomitant use may reduce the efficacy of spironolactone.[10]
Hormonal contraceptives	See Chapters 2 and 3 on hormonal contraception.	See Chapters 2 and 3 on hormonal contraception.

GI, gastrointestinal; NSAIDs: nonsteroidal anti-inflammatory drugs.

MANAGING SIDE EFFECTS

Consult with a provider regarding patient reported side effects.

CLINICAL PEARL BOX 1

METFORMIN SIDE EFFECTS

- Metallic taste in mouth: This affects about three in 100 people.[9]
  - Continue taking the medication as prescribed and symptoms generally will subside after a short time.[9]
- Gastrointestinal complaints
  - Continue taking the medication as prescribed and symptoms generally will subside after a short time.[9] The patient should take metformin with food to reduce symptoms.[9]
  - If symptoms last longer than a few weeks, call provider; a dosage adjustment may be necessary.[9]

CLINICAL PEARL BOX 2

Patients using Spironolactone should avoid potassium supplements, medications that increase the level of serum potassium, and/or foods containing high levels of potassium, including salt substitutes.[10]

SUMMARY

- PCOS occurs in some females as the result of a hormone imbalance in which androgen levels are higher than normal. It embodies a broad range of presentations, but it is generally diagnosed when two of the following are present: anovulation, irregular, or heavy menstrual bleeding, and hyperandrogenism.[1,2]

- In adolescents, combined hormonal contraception is the first line treatment for PCOS symptoms of acne, hirsutism, menstrual irregularities, and for pregnancy prevention.[2,3]

- When the patient is also overweight or obese, lifestyle changes such as a calorie-restricted diet and increased exercise are also first line recommendations. Metformin is often added to the treatment regimen in the setting of metabolic syndrome.[2,3]

- The symptoms of PCOS can be particularly stressful for adolescents and regular follow-up, support, and encouragement by the healthcare team is important to maintain compliance with the treatment regimen in order to improve symptoms.

RELATED PROTOCOLS

■ Chapter 1: Amenorrhea

■ Chapters 2 and 3: Hormonal therapy

References

1. Crouch NS, Allen L. Primary amenorrhea in pediatric and adolescent gynecology practice: clinical evaluation. In: Creighton SM, Belen A, Breech L, Liao LM, eds. *Pediatric and Adolescent Gynecology: A Problem-Base Approach.* New York, NY: Cambridge University Press; 2018:86–87.
2. North American Society for Pediatric and Adolescent Gynecology. NASPAG patient handout: Polycystic ovary syndrome (PCOS). 2019. https://www.naspag .org/page/patienttools
3. Legro RS, Arsianian SA, Ehrmann DA, et al. Diagnosis and treatment of polycystic ovary syndrome: an endocrine society clinical practice guideline. *J Clin Endocrinol Metab.* 2013;98(12):4565–4592. doi:10.1210/jc.2013-2350
4. Martin KA, Anderson RR, Chang RJ, et al. Evaluation and treatment of hirsutism in premenopausal women: an endocrine society clinical practice guideline. *J Clin Endocrinol Metab.* 2018;103(4):1233–1257. doi:10.1210/jc.2018-00241
5. Sam S. Obesity and polycystic ovary syndrome. *Obes Manag.* 2007;3920:69–73. doi:10.1089/obe.2007.0019
6. Smith RA, von Eschenbach AC, Wender R, et al. ACS Prostate Cancer Advisory Committee, ACS Colorectal Cancer Advisory Committee, ACS Endometrial Cancer Advisory Committee. American Cancer Society guidelines for the early detection of cancer: update of early detection guidelines for prostate, colorectal, and endometrial cancers. Also: update 2001–testing for early lung cancer detection. *CA Cancer J Clin.* 2001;51:38–75. doi:10.3322/canjclin.51.1.38
7. Setji TL, Brown AJ. Polycystic ovary syndrome: update on diagnosis and treatment. *Am J Med.* 2014;127(10):912–919. doi:10.1016/j.amjmed.2014.04.017
8. American Diabetes Association. Executive summary: standards of medical care in diabetes-2013. *Diabetes Care.* 2013;36(1):S4–S9. doi:10.2337/dc13-S004
9. *Glucophage* (Package insert). Princeton, NJ: Bristol-Meyers Squibb Co.; 2018.
10. *Aldactone* (Package insert). New York, NY: Pfizer, Inc.; 2018.

16

POSITIVE PREGNANCY TEST
Jane Geyer

INTRODUCTION

Patients often seek advice from a gynecology office after a positive at-home pregnancy test. Pregnancy can be diagnosed by both urine and serum testing. A random urine sample can be taken at any time of the day and most standard home pregnancy kits are usually positive within 7 days after the last missed period.[1] The most sensitive home pregnancy tests can detect pregnancy as early as the first day of a missed period.[2] Serum testing can be positive as early as six days after suspected conception, and is most accurate, as the levels of Beta HcG are generally detectable in the serum before the hormones are detectable in urine.[3,4]

When a patient reports a positive pregnancy test, the nurse should first assess the patient's safety, as some teens may be fearful to notify their partner and/or family members. Finally, because this may result in patient anxiety, it is also important to assess if the patient is having thoughts of hurting herself or committing suicide.

CLINICAL PEARL BOX

Patients with positive pregnancy tests should still always be encouraged to use barrier contraception to help prevent transmission of sexually transmitted infections (STIs).

The patient should be offered a clinic visit to confirm the results and discuss the results with a provider. This visit should occur rather urgently, as confirming a pregnancy early can maximize the time the patient has to consider all options available. The nurse should be familiar with all public health facilities available for teens who may not feel comfortable discussing the results with a guardian present.

The triage nurse should always provide emotional support and educate the patient on healthy pregnancy and red flags.

COMMON PATIENT CONCERNS

- Mixed pregnancy test results
- Prenatal vitamins
- Discontinuing hormonal contraceptives
- Pregnancy symptoms

⊙ KEY QUESTIONS TO ASK

- When was the pregnancy test taken?
- When was the patient's last menstrual cycle (LMP)?
- When was the patient's most recent sexual activity?
- Was the sexual activity consensual?
- Has the patient notified the partner and/or guardian about the positive test?
- Does the patient feel safe at home?
- Is the patient using any type of hormonal birth control?
- Is the patient using prenatal vitamins?
- Is the patient using drugs/alcohol or smoking cigarettes?
- Is the patient having abdominal pain?
- Is the patient having abnormal vaginal bleeding?

TABLE 16.1 Common Patient Concerns Regarding a Positive Pregnancy Test

Common Patient Concerns	Counseling/Nursing Intervention
Mixed pregnancy test results	■ If a patient takes multiple tests and gets both positive and negative results or suspects an error in the result, recommend taking a repeat pregnancy test in 7 days. At-home urine pregnancy tests are usually accurate 7 days after the expected menstrual cycle.[5] ■ For patients with irregular menstrual cycles, recommend a repeat test in 2 weeks. ■ Always offer the patient a clinic visit to confirm the results.
Prenatal vitamins	Recommend the patient start over-the-counter prenatal vitamins. The patient should look for a vitamin with at least 0.4 mg of folic acid to help prevent neural tube defects.[6] Neural tube development occurs during the first few weeks of pregnancy, and closure of the neural tube occurs by 6 weeks of gestation.

(continued)

TABLE 16.1 Common Patient Concerns Regarding a Positive Pregnancy Test (*continued*)

Common Patient Concerns	Counseling/Nursing Intervention
	Patients on certain medications or with a family history of neural tube defects may require higher doses of folic acid.
Birth control	■ Until the pregnancy has been confirmed, advise the patient to continue her hormonal birth control option if it is the pill, patch, or ring. Evidence is lacking in use of the patch or ring during pregnancy; however, the pill has not been shown to have detrimental effects on the pregnancy or fetus.[7] Once the patient has a confirmed pregnancy test in office, the provider can discontinue the hormonal contraceptive option.
	■ If the patient has an arm implant or IUD in place, please assist the patient in making an office visit to discuss removal.
	■ If the patient has been using Medroxyprogesterone acetate, the patient should not receive any further injections until after her delivery.[8,9]
	The nurse should counsel the patient to continue to use barrier contraception regardless of pregnancy status to prevent transmission of STIs.
Pregnancy symptoms	■ The most common symptoms during early pregnancy include amenorrhea, nausea/vomiting, breast tenderness, urinary frequency, and fatigue. Most patients can expect to experience their first pregnancy symptoms between 5–8 weeks of gestation.[10] Pregnancy symptoms ultimately need to be managed by the patient's obstetrics provider so management of common symptoms will not be discussed in this chapter.
	■ Although rare, it is always important to consider the risk of ectopic pregnancy and nonviable pregnancies. Ectopic pregnancy, or implantation outside of the uterine cavity, occurs in approximately 2% of the general population.[11] The most common presenting symptoms include abdominal pain and vaginal bleeding.[11] The symptoms will typically present between 6–8 weeks after the patient's LMP.

IUD, intrauterine device; LMP, last menstrual cycle; STIs, sexually transmitted infections.

➡️ **RED FLAGS**

Safety Concerns: If the patient is in immediate danger, the patient should hang up and call 9-1-1. If the patient is not in immediate danger but is scared to discuss a positive pregnancy result with a guardian or partner, encourage the patient to wait for the office visit to discuss in a safe environment with the provider.

> Note: If the patient is having thoughts of self-harm or suicide, it is important that the nurse identify the patient's current location and whether the patient has a plan. If the patient has a plan and is in immediate danger, the nurse should notify a guardian or someone in the home and contact the police. Teens have a higher risk of completing suicide and most reports of attempted self-harm, medication overdose in particular, occur early on after discovering the pregnancy.[12,13]

Abdominal pain: Abdominal pain during pregnancy may be, although not limited to, a sign of ectopic pregnancy, tubal rupture, or missed abortion in early pregnancy. In the case of ectopic pregnancy, it is usually located in the pelvic region but can present with a wide variety of characteristics and severity.[11] Tubal rupture can occur with ectopic pregnancy and may be associated with an abrupt onset of severe, constant pain, but can also present with more mild, intermittent pain. Given the wide variety of presentation of obstetrical emergencies, the triage nurse should notify a provider immediately and recommend the patient seek evaluation in the ED.

Vaginal bleeding: Bleeding during early pregnancy can be physiologic, or can be a sign of ectopic pregnancy, spontaneous abortion, gestational trophoblastic disease, or a vaginal/uterine pathology. Physiologic bleeding in those with known or suspected bleeding should be a diagnosis of exclusion; therefore, the triage nurse should notify a provider immediately and refer the patient to the ED for assessment.

⬛ SPECIAL POPULATION CONSIDERATIONS

Patients with certain chronic conditions place them at higher risk for certain pregnancy complications, including maternal and fetal death.

TABLE 16.2 Special Population Considerations Regarding a Positive Pregnancy Test

Special Population	Significance	Intervention/Delegation
Teratogenic medication use	The FD has guidelines for medications that assist providers and patients in weighing risks and benefits of medications during pregnancy.	▪ Assist the patient and/or guardian in reviewing and listing out medications for the patient's prenatal office visit.

(continued)

TABLE 16.2 Special Population Considerations Regarding a Positive Pregnancy Test (*continued*)

Special Population	Significance	Intervention/Delegation
	Some common medications that are considered contraindicated in pregnancy include alcohol, anticoagulants, hydantoin, isotretinoin, lithium carbonate, methotrexate, thalidomide,[14] valproate sodium.[14]	■ If the patient is using any high-risk medications, immediately contact a provider.
Bleeding and coagulation disorders	Patients with bleeding disorders may be at higher risk for bleeding complications related to pregnancy or delivery.[15]	■ Patients with congenital bleeding disorders or those on coagulation should discuss their pregnancy risks with their obstetrician. The patient may need to be followed by a MFM. ■ Assist the patient and/or guardian in reviewing and listing out medications for the patient's prenatal office visit. ■ If the patient is using any high-risk medications, such as anticoagulants, immediately contact a provider. ■ Review heavy bleeding precautions with patient and signs of missed AB.
CVD	Due to the hemodynamic changes in the cardiovascular system that occur during pregnancy, patients with underlying cardiac disease may be at a higher risk for pregnancy complications and mortality.[16] The WHO has classified heart and valvular conditions by Category I-IV, with class IV having the highest risk of morbidity and mortality.[17]	■ Patients with CVD should discuss their pregnancy risks with their obstetrician. The patient may need to be followed by a MFM. ■ Assist the patient and/or guardian in reviewing and listing out medications for the patient's prenatal office visit. ■ If the patient is using any high-risk medications, such as anticoagulants, immediately contact a provider.

(*continued*)

TABLE 16.2 Special Population Considerations Regarding a Positive Pregnancy Test (*continued*)

Special Population	Significance	Intervention/Delegation
CKD	Patients with mild CKD are likely to have favorable pregnancy outcomes.[18] Patients with moderate to severe CKD are more likely to experience worsening of renal dysfunction and adverse pregnancy complications such as preeclampsia and preterm delivery.[18]	▪ Patients with CKD should discuss their pregnancy risks with their obstetrician. The patient will need to be followed by an MFM. ▪ Assist the patient and/or guardian in reviewing and listing out medications for the patient's prenatal office visit.
Seizure disorder	Multiple medications used for the treatment of epilepsy can be teratogenic to the patient and the fetus.[14]	▪ Assist the patient and/or guardian in reviewing and listing out medications for the patient's prenatal office visit. ▪ If the patient is using any high-risk medications, such as anticoagulants, immediately contact a provider.
Sickle cell disease	Females with sickle cell disease can have increased pain crises during pregnancy. They may also be at a higher risk of preterm labor, preeclampsia, pulmonary complications, and infection than those without the disease.[19]	▪ Patients with sickle cell disease should discuss their pregnancy risks with their obstetrician. The patient may need to be followed by an MFM.
SLE	SLE patients are known to have higher risk of pregnancy-related complications including but are not limited to: Preterm labor, fetal growth restriction, pre-eclampsia, eclampsia.[20] Pregnancy can increase the risk of VTE, thrombocytopenia, infection, HTN, and postpartum hemorrhage in patients with SLE.[21]	▪ Pregnant SLE patients should always be followed by a maternal–fetal medicine specialist. Please contact a provider for a referral. ▪ Assist the patient and/or guardian in reviewing and listing out medications for the patient's prenatal office visit. ▪ If a patient is using a high-risk medication, such as anticoagulants or methotrexate, immediately contact a provider.

AB, abortion; CKD, chronic kidney disease; CVD, cardiovascular disease; HTN, hypertension; MFM, maternal–fetal medicine specialist; SLE, systemic lupus erythematosus; VTE, venous thromboembolism; WHO, World Health Organization.

SUMMARY

The nurse may be the first healthcare provider notified when a patient takes a positive pregnancy test. It is important for the gynecology nurse to be familiar with early obstetrical emergencies and red flags. The nurse should always assess the patient's safety, and can provide guidance and education on early lifestyle modifications the patient may need to make as well as provide advice about going to the ED for a higher level of care if warranted.

RELATED PROTOCOLS

▨ Refer to Food and Drug Administration (FDA) guidelines for medication use in pregnancy.

▨ The nurse should be familiar with the facility policy in case a patient endorses experiencing suicidal thoughts or safety concerns.

References

1. Ayala A, Bustos H, Aguilar R. Daily rhythm of serum human chorionic gonadotropin and human chorionic somatomammotropin in normal pregnancy. *Int J Gynaecol Obstet*. 1984;22(3):173. doi:10.1016/0020-7292(84)90001-8
2. Cole L. The utility of six over-the-counter (home) pregnancy tests. *Clin Chem Lab Med*. 2011;49(8):1317. doi:10.1515/CCLM.2011.211
3. Braunstein G, Rasor J, Danzer H, Adler D, Wade M. Serum human chorionic gonadotropin levels throughout normal pregnancy. *Am J Obstet Gynecol*. 1976;126(6):678. doi:10.1016/0002-9378(76)90518-4
4. O'Connor R, Bibro C, Pegg P, Bouzoukis J. The comparative sensitivity and specificity of serum and urine HCG determinations in the ED. *Am J Emerg Med*. 1993;11(4):434. doi:10.1016/0735-6757(93)90186-F
5. Wilcox AJ, Baird D, Dunson D, McChesney R, Weinberg C. Natural limits of pregnancy testing in relation to the expected menstrual period. *JAMA*. 2001;286(14):1759. doi:10.1001/jama.286.14.1759
6. Berry R, Li Z, Erickson, J, et al. Prevention of neural-tube defects with folic acid in China. China-U.S. collaborative project for neural tube defect prevention. *N Engl J Med*. 1999;341(20):1485–1490. doi:10.1056/NEJM199911113412001
7. Bracken MB. Oral contraception and congenital malformations in offspring: a review and meta-analysis of the prospective studies. *Obstet Gynecol*. 1990;76:552–557
8. Gray R, Pardthaisong T. In utero exposure to steroid contraceptives and survival during infancy. *Am J Epidemiol*. 1991;134:804–811. doi:10.1093/oxfordjournals.aje.a116153
9. Pardthaisong T, Gray RH. In utero exposure to steroid contraceptives and outcome of pregnancy. *Am J Epidemiol*. 1991;134:795–803. doi:10.1093/oxfordjournals.aje.a116152
10. Sayle AE, Wilcox A, Weinberg C, Baird D. A prospective study of the onset of symptoms of pregnancy. *J Clin Epidemiol*. 2002;55(7):676. doi:10.1016/S0895-4356(02)00402-X

11. Alkatout I, Honemeyer U, Strauss A, et al. Clinical diagnosis and treatment of ectopic pregnancy. *Obstet Gynecol Surv.* 2013;68(8):571. doi:10.1097/OGX.0b013e31829cdbeb

12. Lindahl V, Pearson J, Colpe L. Prevalence of suicidality during pregnancy and the postpartum. *Arch Womens Ment Health.* 2005;8(2):77. doi:10.1007/s00737-005-0080-1

13. Czeizel A, Tímár L, Susánszky E. Timing of suicide attempts by self-poisoning during pregnancy and pregnancy outcomes. *Int J Gynaecol Obstet.* 1999;65(1):39. doi:10.1016/S0020-7292(99)00007-7

14. Friedman J, Polifka, J. *Teratogenic effects of drugs: a Resource for clinicians (TERIS).* 2nd ed. Baltimore, MD: John Hopkins University Press; 2000.

15. Kadir R, Lee C, Sabin C, Pollard D, Economides D. Pregnancy in women with von Willebrand's disease or factor XI deficiency. *Br J Obstet Gynaecol.* 1998;105(3): 314–321. doi:10.1111/j.1471-0528.1998.tb10093.x

16. Thorne S, MacGregor A, Nelson-Piercy C. Risks of contraception and pregnancy in heart disease. *Heart.* 2006;92(10):1520–1525. doi:10.1136/hrt.2006.095240

17. European Society of Gynecology (ESG), Association for European Paediatric Cardiology (AEPC), German Society for Gender Medicine (DGesGM), et al. ESC Guidelines on the management of cardiovascular diseases during pregnancy: the task force on the management of cardiovascular diseases during pregnancy of the European Society of Cardiology (ESC). *Eur Heart J.* 2011;32(24):3147. doi:10.1093/eurheartj/ehr194

18. Hladunewich M. Chronic kidney disease and pregnancy. *Semin Neophrol.* 2017; 37(4):337–346. doi:10.1016/j.semnephrol.2017.05.005

19. Sun P, Wilburn W, Raynor B, Jamieson D. Sickle cell disease in pregnancy: twenty years of experience at Grady Memorial Hospital, Atlanta, Georgia. *Am J Obstet Gynecol.* 2001;184(6):1127–1130. doi:10.1067/mob.2001.115477

20. Clowse M, Jamison M, Myers E, James A. A national study of the complications of lupus in pregnancy. *Am J Obstet Gynecol.* 2008;199(2):127.e1-6. doi:10.1016/j.ajog.2008.03.012

21. Yasmeen S, Wilkins E, Field N, Sheikh R, Gilbert W. Pregnancy outcomes in women with systemic lupus erythematosus. *J Matern Fetal Med.* 2001;10(2):91. doi:10.1080/jmf.10.2.91.96

17

POSTOPERATIVE CONCERNS
Jennifer Bercaw-Pratt

INTRODUCTION

The two most common types of surgeries that pediatric and adolescent gyne-cology providers perform are abdominal and vaginal surgeries. These sur-geries can vary in complexity from an exam under anesthesia to a complex reconstructive surgery. This chapter will focus on the common postoperative complaints for both abdominal and vaginal surgeries.

Surgical patients will frequently call with complaints of postoperative pain and/or requesting pain medications. Many of these calls are related to a need to reorder medications. However, some of the calls will be for new-onset pain or poorly controlled pain. It is important to know the location of the patient's pain as it may or may not be at the surgical site.[1] For example, patients will frequently complain of shoulder pain following laparoscopy due to stimu-lation of the diaphragm from the residual carbon dioxide gas used to insuf-flate the abdomen during surgery. Inquiring about the severity of the pain is important, as severe pain is treated differently than mild pain.[2] With further questioning, nurses can help determine if the postoperative pain is a normal part of the healing process or alternatively due to bleeding (hematoma), local infections (cellulitis/abscess), musculoskeletal issues, and more serious sys-temic concerns (peritonitis, pneumonia).[1]

Another problem surgical patients frequently call with is postoperative fever. Most postop fevers are not found to have documented causes.[3] When evaluating patient for a postop fever, it is important to inquire about other associated symptoms as this will often will signal the underlying cause. The most common reasons for postop fever include wound infection, urinary tract infection (associated with urinary frequency, urgency, dysuria, and/or costovertebral angle [CVA] tenderness), respiratory infection such as pneu-monia (associated with cough), and thromboembolism (associated with leg pain or swelling, chest pain, and/or shortness of breath).[1,4] The timing of fever is important to establish as early onset of fever is less likely to be infec-tious in etiology.[1,4]

Another common concern for postop patients may be related to the surgical incision. Most of these patients will have minor oozing from the surgical site. Minor oozing is typically is seen on the outer wound dressings and may be related to fibrin production, which is part of normal wound healing. Symptoms that are concerning for a more serious wound complication (seroma, hematoma, and fistula) include substantial amounts of serous, serosanguinous, or bloody discharge from the surgical site.[4] Additional symptoms of a wound infection include purulent or foul-smelling discharge from the surgical site with erythema, induration, and tenderness of the surrounding tissues.[4]

Abdominal distension and nausea/vomiting postoperatively can be due to ileus and/or bowel obstruction.[3,5] Ileus usually occurs with distension in the first 2 to 3 days after surgery versus obstruction, which is abdominal cramping with delayed onset 5 to 7 days after surgery. Constipation is a common concern after surgery as well.[4] This is usually related to narcotic medications utilized for pain control postoperatively. It is important to establish when the patient last had a bowel movement prior to surgery and after surgery. Additionally, some patients may have been feeling ill prior to surgery and may not have been eating well. In this situation, it is not uncommon for some postoperative patients to not have a bowel movement; however, they should have signs of bowel function, which includes gas passage. If they are tolerating liquids and foods, that is always a good sign. However, if they are bloated, ensuring they are drinking plenty of fluids, eating fruits and vegetables, and taking a stool softener are important reminders for the patient.

Vaginal bleeding or discharge may be a concern for patients who have undergone a vaginal procedure. Some bleeding and discharge, especially if creams are being applied, may be normal. If they are having worsening pain, swelling, foul-smelling discharge, or heavy bleeding enough to soak one pad in an hour, they should be seen by a surgeon.[3]

CLINICAL PEARL BOX

There are patients with medical comorbidities that place the patient at higher risk for postoperative complications. Some examples of common comorbidities seen in the pediatric and adolescent gynecology practice include obesity, diabetes, medical therapy with steroids, and anti-coagulation.

COMMON PATIENT CONCERNS

- Pain
- Fever
- Wound concerns
- Nausea/vomiting
- Vaginal bleeding

⊙ KEY QUESTIONS TO ASK

All postoperative concerns

▪ What operation did the patient have, and when was it performed?

Pain concerns

▪ Where is the patient's pain, and how severe is the pain?
▪ Are there any other symptoms associated with the pain, such as dysuria, vomiting, bloating, or diarrhea?
▪ What pain medication, if any, is the patient taking now?

Fever concerns

▪ Does the patient have a fever? How high is the fever?
▪ Are there any other symptoms associated with the fever, such as wound concerns, leg pain, back pain, cough, or dysuria?

Wound concerns

▪ What type of discharge is seen coming from the surgical site? Serous, serosanguinous, bloody, or purulent?
▪ Are there associated skin changes such as erythema, induration, or tenderness surrounding the surgical site?

Nausea/vomiting

▪ Is the patient able to keep down liquids?
▪ Is the patient passing gas and/or having bowel movements?

For vaginal bleeding concerns

▪ How much vaginal bleeding is the patient experiencing? When did it start? Does the patient have associated symptoms of anemia such as dizziness?

PATIENT ASSESSMENT

TABLE 17.1 Acute Symptoms Commonly Experienced After Gynecologic Surgery

Acute Symptoms	Intervention/Delegation	Commonly Prescribed Medicine
Fever	Inquire about associated symptoms to relay to the surgeon.	Acetaminophen
Dysuria	Inquire about associated symptoms to relay to the surgeon.	The physician may consider prescribing an antibiotic.

(continued)

TABLE 17.1 Acute Symptoms Commonly Experienced After Gynecologic Surgery (*continued*)

Acute Symptoms	Intervention/Delegation	Commonly Prescribed Medicine
Cough	Inquire about associated symptoms to relay to the surgeon.	N/A
Chest pain	Requires emergent evaluation.	N/A
Shortness of breath	Requires emergent evaluation.	N/A
Pain	Inquire about associated symptoms to relay to the surgeon.	The surgeon may choose to recommend acetaminophen, NSAIDs, or narcotic pain medication.
Wound bleeding	Inquire about associated symptoms to relay to the surgeon. The patient can consider changing the wound dressing.	N/A
Erythema at the wound	Inquire about associated symptoms to relay to the surgeon. The patient can consider marking the periphery of the incision for closer monitoring.	N/A
Nausea/vomiting	Inquire about associated symptoms to relay to the surgeon.	The surgeon may choose to recommend an anti-emetic such as promethazine or ondansetron.
Constipation	Inquire about when patient last ate or drank. Inquire about last bowel movement prior to and after surgery. Inquire about passage of gas. Inquire about use of stool softeners.	The surgeon may choose to recommend stool softeners or anti-gas medications.
Vaginal bleeding	Quantify the amount of bleeding to relay to the surgeon.	N/A

NSAIDs, nonsteroidal anti-inflammatory drugs.

➡ RED FLAGS

Deep vein thrombosis (DVT): These are common in postsurgical patients, especially in the setting of a long surgery. Although DVTs originate in the leg or the pelvis, they may travel to the pulmonary artery. This may lead to a life-threatening pulmonary embolus. Both DVT and pulmonary embolism (PE) can be difficult to diagnose, so it is important to have a high level of suspicion when patients present with symptoms in the immediate postoperative period. Symptoms of DVT include leg pain and/or leg swelling that is unresponsive to acetaminophen or nonsteroidal anti-inflammatory drugs (NSAIDs), while a pulmonary embolus can present with chest pain or tightness, rapid heart rate, and shortness of breath.[4]

Pneumonia: This is another serious postoperative complication. These patients typically report a cough in association with fever, shortness of breath, and purulent sputum.[3]

Pelvic abscess: A pelvic abscess can develop in patients undergoing intra-abdominal or vaginal surgery where the abdominal cavity was entered. The symptoms that are concerning for pelvic abscess include fever and abdominal pain/pelvic pain occurring late in the recovery period (typically after postop day 3).[3,4]

◉ SPECIAL POPULATION CONSIDERATIONS

There are patients with medical comorbidities that place the patient at higher risk for postoperative complications.

- Obesity: Patients with obesity are two to three times more likely to have perioperative death and morbidity. This is due to several reasons including, but not limited to, elevated risk for cardiopulmonary complications, wound complications, and venous thrombosis.[4]
- Diabetes: Patients with diabetes are at increased risk of impaired wound healing due to large and small blood vessel disease, which impairs delivery of oxygen to surgical site, and increased infection due to impaired immunity.[6]
- Medical comorbidities requiring chronic use of steroids: Patients who require chronic use of steroids have delayed wound healing and increased rates of wound infections.[6]
- Anti-coagulated patients: Patients who are on anti-coagulation may have increased acute and delayed bleeding at the surgical site.[1]

SUMMARY

■ Patients will frequently call during the postoperative period.

■ It is important to distinguish which symptoms are part of the normal healing process or alternatively due to a postoperative complication.

RELATED PROTOCOLS

■ Chapter 21: Urinary Concerns

■ Chapter 8: Bleeding Concerns

■ Chapter 13: Acute Pelvic Pain

References

1. Adams G, Bresnick S. *On Call Surgery*, vol. 2. Philadelphia, PA: W. B. Saunders; 2001.
2. Wong M, Morris S, Wang K, et al. Managing post-operative pain after minimally invasive gynecologic surgery in the era of opiod surgery. *J Minim Invasive Gynecol.* 2018;25(7):1165–1178. doi:10.1016/j.jmig.2017.09.016
3. Jones H, Rock J, eds. *Te Linde's Operative Gynecology*, vol. 9. Philadelphia, PA: Lippincott Williams & Wilkins; 2003.
4. Quick C, Reed J, Harper S, et al. eds. *Essential Surgery: Problems, Diagnosis and Management*, vol. 5. London, England: Churchill Livingstone Elsevier; 2014.
5. Sanfilippo F, Spoletini G. Perspectives on the post-operative Ileus. *Curr Med Res Opin.* 2015;31(4):675–676. doi:10.1185/03007995.2015.1027184.
6. Sutton J, Beckwith M, Johnson B, et al., eds. *The Mont Reid Surgical Handbook*, vol. 7. Philadelphia, PA: Elsevier; 2018.

18

PRIMARY OVARIAN INSUFFICIENCY
Kara Bendle and Deborah Morse

INTRODUCTION

Primary ovarian insufficiency (POI) is characterized by a serum follicle-stimulating hormone (FSH) concentration in the menopausal range.[1] The development of POI is often spontaneous in an otherwise healthy patient and in most presentations, the cause of POI cannot be specifically identified.[1] The etiology of POI can be genetic, autoimmune, idiopathic or iatrogenic/secondary to other medical conditions.[2,3] Ovarian injury may occur in patients with a history of receiving chemotherapy and/or radiation resulting in ovarian insufficiency.[4]

Symptoms associated with POI are related to estrogen deficiency and may include primary or secondary amenorrhea, lack of or arrest of development of secondary sexual characteristics, hot flashes, night sweats, sleep disturbances, vaginal dryness, or dyspareunia.[1,2,5]

Recommended interventions may include hormone replacement therapy (HRT), calcium and vitamin D supplementation, and weight-bearing exercise[1] The purpose of HRT in the setting of POI is to provide physiologic levels of hormones in order to support bone, cardiovascular, and sexual health, along with symptomatic relief. Girls who present before secondary sexual characteristics have begun developing will likely need different interventions than those who present after pubertal development is complete. A referral to a practitioner with expertise in pubertal growth and development for hormonal therapy may be recommended.[5]

It is important to understand that the sudden, spontaneous nature of the presentation of POI can elicit a very profound emotional response in patients and families. Referral to counseling and peer support resources, as well as long-term follow up by a multidisciplinary team, is essential to avoid psychological distress, anxiety, and low self-esteem.[1,2,5] Management of POI should address both the physical and emotional aspects of the condition.

CLINICAL PEARL BOX

It is important to note that hormone replacement therapy (HRT) may not work effectively for contraception in patients with POI.[1] If a patient is sexually active, the nurse should recommend a clinic visit for the patient to discuss a potential intrauterine device (IUD).[1] The nurse should advise all sexually active teens to use condoms.

COMMON PATIENT CONCERNS

- Anxiety/Depression
- Bone health
- Cardiovascular health
- Contraception
- Hormonal therapy
- Hot flashes and/or night sweats
- Menstrual irregularities
- Options for becoming a parent
- Sexual health
- Vaginal dryness

(O) KEY QUESTIONS TO ASK

- Is the patient menarchal? If so, how often is the patient having menses? When was the patient's first menstrual period? When was the patient's last menstrual period (LMP)?
- Is the patient using hormonal replacement therapy, such as pills or a transdermal patch? If so, is the patient adherent to the treatment?
- Does the patient have any hot flashes, night sweats, and/or vaginal dryness?
- Is the patient sexually active?

PATIENT ASSESSMENT

TABLE 18.1 Acute Symptoms of Premature Ovarian Insufficiency

Acute Symptoms	Intervention/Delegation	Commonly Prescribed Medicine
Hot flashes/night sweats	▦ Reassure the patient that symptoms should diminish once physiologic levels of estrogen are achieved. ▦ Encourage compliance with prescribed medications. ▦ If patient reports symptoms despite medication compliance or displeasure with current medication regimen, consult provider or schedule office visit.[5]	▦ Estradiol
Menstrual irregularities	▦ Schedule an office visit for evaluation. ▦ Encourage compliance with prescribed medications. ▦ Encourage home pregnancy test if sexually active.[1] ▦ Recommend keeping a menstrual calendar.[1]	▦ Estradiol ▦ Medroxyprogesterone acetate
Vaginal dryness/dyspareunia	▦ Reassure the patient that symptoms should diminish once physiologic levels of estrogen are achieved. ▦ Encourage compliance with prescribed medications. ▦ If patient reports symptoms despite medication compliance or displeasure with current medication regimen, consult provider or schedule office visit.[5]	▦ Estradiol ▦ Lubricant

TABLE 18.2 Chronic Symptoms of Premature Ovarian Insufficiency

Chronic Symptoms	Intervention/Delegation	Commonly Prescribed Medicine
Anxiety/depression	Help the patient identify sources of emotional support. Refer to counseling and/or peer support group. Reassure the patient that these feelings are common for young women receiving this diagnosis. Discuss strategies to share diagnosis with family, friends, and partners.[1,5] For parental anxiety/depression: Recommend the parent seek counseling in order to address their reasonable and expected feelings of grief and loss and learn techniques to better support their daughter. Assess their knowledge and understanding of the medical information. Encourage calmness, confidence, and positivity.[1,2,5,6]	
Bone health/osteoporosis	Encourage compliance with medication regimen. Coordinate bone mineral density testing as ordered by provider.[1,5] Recommend regular weight-bearing exercise such as walking or jogging.[1,5]	Calcium Vitamin D[1]
Cardiovascular issues	Encourage healthy diet.[1] Encourage maintenance of a healthy BMI.[1] Discourage tobacco use.[5] Coordinate screening for cardiovascular risk factors as ordered by provider.[1] For DVT-related concerns, reassure the patient that maintaining physiologic rather than elevated estrogen levels decreases risk. Use of the transdermal patch as opposed to oral pills avoids the first pass effect on the liver and further reduces the risk of developing a thromboembolism.[1,5]	Estradiol transdermal patch[1]

(continued)

TABLE 18.2 Chronic Symptoms of Premature Ovarian Insufficiency (*continued*)

Chronic Symptoms	Intervention/Delegation	Commonly Prescribed Medicine
Contraception	Stress that medication regimens for POI do not provide birth control.	Hormonal contraception
	Review the variable nature of ovarian function as some patients may spontaneously ovulate.[7]	Barrier contraception
	If a patient is sexually active, recommend use of barrier methods and recommend an office visit to discuss birth control, such as an intrauterine device.	
	Advise the patient to keep a menstrual calendar and taking a pregnancy test if a period is late.[1]	
Hormone replacement therapy	Reassure the patient that adherence to medication regimens can help reduce negative long-term health concerns.	Estradiol Medroxyprogesterone acetate
	Review objectives of medication regimens: maintaining physiologic hormone levels, providing symptom relief, and protecting bone, uterine, and cardiovascular health.[1,5]	
Menstrual bleeding complaints	Assess if medications have been used as prescribed (correct cyclic progesterone schedule, correct patch schedule, difficulties getting patch to adhere, etc.).	Estradiol Medroxyprogesterone acetate
	If patient has been compliant with medication use as prescribed and symptoms persist, consult provider or schedule office visit.	
Options for becoming a parent	Reassure the patient that options exist should she desire to be a mom in the future, i.e., adoption, foster parenthood, egg donation, embryo donation, as well as experimental protocols to potentiate fertility. Ask provider if measuring anti-Mullerian hormone as a marker of reproductive potential is appropriate. Coordinate referral to a reproductive endocrinology and infertility specialist when appropriate.[1,2,5]	

(*continued*)

TABLE 18.2 Chronic Symptoms of Premature Ovarian Insufficiency (*continued*)

Chronic Symptoms	Intervention/Delegation	Commonly Prescribed Medicine
Sexual health	Discuss compliance with medication regimen. Review role of medications in maintaining optimal uterine and vaginal health.[5]	

BMI, body mass index; DVT, deep vein thrombosis.

➡ RED FLAGS

Persistent patient reports of symptoms of low estrogen levels, such as **hot flashes, night sweats, sleep disturbances, or dyspareunia,** might suggest medication noncompliance. It is essential for patients with POI to be compliant with long-term HRT. Encourage medication regimen compliance and facilitate scheduling follow-up visits to establish continuity of care and monitor HRT.

TABLE 18.3 Special Population Considerations for Premature Ovarian Insufficiency

Chronic Condition	Special Intervention/ Delegation	Commonly Prescribed Medicine
Turner Syndrome—affects 25–50 per 100,000 females. Multiple organ systems are involved necessitating a multidisciplinary model of care and can be associated with short stature, delayed puberty, cognitive deficits, and infertility.[2,8]	Refer to provider to start hormone replacement therapy between 11 and 12 years of age.[8] Refer to provider to discuss fertility preservation options early, since the chances of spontaneous conception decrease rapidly with age.[8] Assess for use of contraception if sexually active. Coordinate cardiac imaging as ordered by provider before considering pregnancy, at the appearance of hypertension, and when transitioning from pediatric to adult care.[5,8] Coordinate referral to reproductive endocrinology and infertility specialist prior to considering pregnancy. Women with Turner Syndrome have an increased cardiovascular risk, including a high risk of aortic rupture.[8]	Estrogen replacement[8] Progesterone replacement[8]

(continued)

TABLE 18.3 Special Population Considerations for Premature Ovarian Insufficiency (*continued*)

Chronic Condition	Special Intervention/ Delegation	Commonly Prescribed Medicine
Cancer treatment, late effects of therapy, and survivorship	Predicting the extent of reproductive impairment and the window of fertility for family planning has proven challenging.[4] There is limited data on how to best use ovarian reserve markers such as AMH in counseling young cancer survivors.[4] Schedule fertility preservation counseling **as soon as possible before** chemotherapy or radiation is initiated.[4] Fertility and maternalfetal specialist counseling is recommended in survivorship.[4] Have patient/parent/guardian give authorization to obtain previous medical records. Assess patient questions/goals.	Estrogen replacement[2] Progesterone replacement[2]

AMH, anti-mullerian hormone.

TABLE 18.4 Commonly Prescribed Medicines for Treatment of Premature Ovarian Insufficiency

Medicine	Common Side Effects	Common Interactions
PROGESTERONE REPLACEMENT Commonly prescribed pills: Medroxyprogesterone (Prescribed after breast maturity has been achieved which will	Breast tenderness Breakthrough bleeding Spotting (minor vaginal bleeding) Irregular periods Amenorrhea Depression	**It is important to use medications as prescribed.** No formal pharmacokinetic drug interaction studies have been conducted with medroxyprogesterone and/or LNG-IUD.

(*continued*)

TABLE 18.4 Commonly Prescribed Medicines for Treatment of Premature Ovarian Insufficiency (*continued*)

Medicine	Common Side Effects	Common Interactions
be determined by the provider—if pills used, they are prescribed cyclically, often for the first 12 days of every month).[1] **Commonly prescribed LNG-IUD**	Thromboembolic disorders[9] Additional possible adverse reactions to LNG-IUS: Abdominal pain Vaginal discharge[9]	HIV protease inhibitors, nonnucleoside reverse transcriptase inhibitors. May change serum concentration of progesterone.[10]
ESTROGEN REPLACEMENT **Commonly prescribed:** **Transdermal or oral estradiol formulations**	Headache Breast pain Irregular vaginal bleeding or spotting Stomach/abdominal cramps, bloating Nausea and vomiting Hair loss Libido changes High blood pressure Gallbladder disease Thromboembolic disorders Hypercalcemia[11]	Inducers of CYP3A4 such as St. John's Wort, phenobarbital, carbamazepine, and rifampin may reduce plasma concentrations of estrogens, possibly resulting in a decrease in therapeutic effect.[12] Inhibitors of CYP3A4 such as erythromycin, clarithromycin, ketoconazole, itraconazole, ritonavir, and grapefruit juice may increase plasma concentrations of estrogen.[12]
Vitamin D	Side effects are uncommon at recommended doses.[13] In high doses: Gastrointestinal symptoms: nausea, vomiting, weight loss, metallic taste Fatigue Headache Polyuria Hallucinations Dysrhythmias Muscle/bone pain[13]	

(*continued*)

TABLE 18.4 Commonly Prescribed Medicines for Treatment of Premature Ovarian Insufficiency (*continued*)

Medicine	Common Side Effects	Common Interactions
Calcium	Gastrointestinal symptoms: constipation, belching, gas, nausea/vomiting, loss of appetite, unusual weight loss Mental/mood changes Bone/muscle pain Headaches Increased thirst/urination Weakness and fatigue[13]	

LNG-IUD, levonorgestrel releasing intrauterine device.

MANAGING SIDE EFFECTS

It is important to instruct patients to track any signs or symptoms and to adhere to medication regimens as prescribed. Patients and caregivers should be instructed that medication regimens can be altered and changed if adverse side effects occur or if they have difficulty/displeasure with using a particular regimen.[10]

SUMMARY

POI is a long-term medical condition requiring an interdisciplinary approach in order to promote optimal reproductive, bone, cardiovascular, and emotional health.[1,2,5]

RELATED PROTOCOLS

- ■ Chapters 2 and 3: Hormonal therapy
- ■ Chapter 1: Amenorrhea

References

1. Nelson LM. Primary ovarian insufficiency. *N Engl J Med*. 2009;360(6):606–614. doi:10.1056/NEJMcp0808697
2. Gordon CM, Kanaoka T, Nelson LM. Update on primary ovarian insufficiency in adolescents. *Curr Opin Pediatr*. 2015;27:511–515. doi:10.1097/MOP.0000000000000236
3. Kanj RV, Ofei-Tenkorang NA, Altaye M, Gordon CM. Evaluation and management of primary ovarian insufficiency in adolescents and young adults. *J Pediatr Adolesc Gynecol*. 2018;31(1);13–18. doi:10.1016/j.jpag.2017.07.005

4. Appiah LA, Davies MC. Late effects of childhood cancer in pediatric and adolescent gynecology practice. In: Creighton SM, Belen A, Breech L, Liao LM, eds. *Pediatric and Adolescent Gynecology: A Problem-Based Approach*. New York, NY: Cambridge University Press, 2018;132–138.

5. American College of Obstetricians and Gynecologists. ACOG committee opinion no. 605: primary ovarian insufficiency in adolescents and young women. *Obstet Gynecol*. 2014;123:193–197. doi:10.1097/01.AOG.0000451757.51964.98

6. Covington SN, Hillard PJ, Sterling EW, Nelson, LM. A family systems approach to primary ovarian insufficiency. *J Pediatr Adolesc Gynecol*. 2011;24(3):137–141. doi:10.1016/j.jpag.2010.12.004

7. Van Kasteren YM, Schoemaker J. Premature ovarian failure: a systematic review on therapeutic interventions to restore ovarian function and achieve pregnancy. *Hum Reprod Update*. 1999;5:483–492. doi:10.1093/humupd/5.5.483

8. Gravholt CH, Andersen NH, Conway GS, et al. Clinical practice guidelines for the care of girls and women with Turner syndrome: proceedings from the 2016 Cincinnati international turner syndrome meeting. *Eur J Endocrinol*. 2017;177(3): G1–G70. doi:10.1530/EJE-17-0430

9. *Provera® (Package Insert)*. New York, NY: Pfizer; 2007.

10. *Mirena® (Package Insert)*. Whippany, NJ: Bayer Healthcare Pharmaceuticals, Inc.; 2017.

11. Adams M, Holland N, Urban C. Drugs for disorders and conditions of the female reproductive system. In: Adams M, Holland N, Urban C, eds. *Pharmacology for Nurses: A Pathophysiologic Approach*. 5th ed. Upper Saddle River, NJ: Pearson Education, Inc., 2017; 782–792.

12. *Vivelle-dot® (Package Insert)*. East Hanover, NJ: Novartis Pharmaceuticals Corporation; 2017.

13. Adams M, Holland N, Urban C. Drugs for nutritional disorders. In: Adams M, Holland N, Urban C eds. *Pharmacology for Nurses: A Pathophysiologic Approach*. 5th ed. Upper Saddle River, NJ: Pearson Education, Inc., 2017; 716–717.

19

STD EXPOSURE
Jessica Ginn

INTRODUCTION

Common sexually transmitted infections (STIs) include HIV, chlamydia, gonorrhea, syphilis, herpes simplex virus (HSV), human papillomavirus (HPV), trichomoniasis, and hepatitis viruses. STI exposure occurs when a person has had a sexual partner with an STI. Untreated STIs can lead to upper genital tract infections, infertility, chronic pelvic pain, and chronic infections with hepatitis viruses and HIV. HPV viruses can lead to genital warts and cancer, such as cervical cancers and oral cancers.[1]

HIV is a virus that progressively depletes CD4 T-lymphocytes, resulting in life-threatening immunodeficiency. The late stage of the infection is called AIDS and usually develops over months to years. A person with acute HIV infection is highly contagious, although he or she may have negative HIV testing during this time.[2]

Chlamydia trachomatis (chlamydia) is an STI that can cause permanent damage to a women's reproductive tract.[3] It is the most common cause of bacterial sexualyl transmitted infections.[4] The prevalence is highest in people 24 years of age or younger. Screening annually is recommended for all women under the age of 25 years and for older women with a new sex partner, more than one sex partner, a sex partner with concurrent partners, and/or a sex partner with an STI.[2]

Neisseria gonorrhoeae (gonorrhea) is an STI that can be seen in the genitals, rectum, or throat.[5] It is the second most commonly reported STI following chlamydia. Screening annually is recommended for all women under the age of 25 years and for older women with a new sex partner, more than one sex partner, a sex partner with concurrent partners, or a sex partner with an STI.[2]

Syphilis is a bacterial infection caused by *Treponema pallidum* that can cause systemic symptoms. The disease has three stages: primary syphilis, secondary syphilis, and tertiary syphilis. Latent syphilis occurs when the patient does not have symptoms of syphilis; however, *Treponema pallidum* is detected on serologic testing. Early latent syphilis occurs when latent syphilis was acquired within the last year. Patients should be evaluated for syphilis if they have had a sexual partner with syphilis. Anybody with primary and secondary syphilis should also be tested for HIV.[2]

Genital herpes is caused by the HSV type 1 or type 2. HSV is transmitted by contact with HSV in lesions, mucosal surfaces, genital secretions, or oral secretions. Transmission can occur even when the infected partner does not have visible lesions. The average incubation period is 4 days after exposure. The risk of HSV transmission to a partner can be reduced by avoiding sexual activity during an outbreak, condom use, and suppressive antiviral therapy. Screening for HSV-1 and HSV-2 is not recommended for the general population.[6]

Forty different strains of HPV can infect the genital area. HPV types 16 and 18 are more likely to cause cervical, vulvar, vaginal, anal, and oropharyngeal cancers. HPV types 6 and 11 are more likely to cause genital warts. Routine cervical cancer screening should be performed starting at age 21 with cytology, and HPV testing should be reserved for very selected cases.[2]

Trichomonas vaginalis (trichomoniasis) is a nonviral STI caused by a protozoan parasite. It is easily transmitted through penile-vaginal intercourse.[2] Trichomoniasis infection can increase the risk of getting other STIs.[7]

The hepatitis B virus (HBV) is a virus that causes hepatitis B liver infections. The incubation period is between 6 weeks and 6 months from the time of exposure. Transmission of HBV occurs by percutaneous or mucous membrane exposure to HBV-infected blood or body fluids that contain HBV.[2] Most HBV infections will resolve own their own, however, some develop into chronic infection.[8]

CLINICAL PEARL BOX

Patients should always be educated on how to protect themselves from sexually transmitted infections (STIs). Patient counseling should encourage the use of condoms. It is also important to inform patients that hormonal contraceptive options do not protect against STIs.

COMMON PATIENT CONCERNS

- The patient may be concerned about the stigma associated with STIs. Providing patients with information about screenings, symptoms, treatment, and how it will affect the patient's overall health may help to relieve stress.
- The patient may be concerned about how to protect themselves from STIs. Patient counseling should encourage the use of condoms.

(O) KEY QUESTIONS TO ASK

Potential Exposure to STI

- Have you had a sexual partner with a diagnosed STI? If so, which STI?
- When was your last sexual activity with an individual with an STI?
- Have you had a new sexual partner, multiple sexual partners, or a sex partner with concurrent partners?
- Have you had oral, anal, or vaginal sex?
- Are you having any symptoms such as vaginal discharge, ulcers on your genitals, pelvic pain, or rectal pain?

PATIENT ASSESSMENT

TABLE 19.1 Common Symptoms of Sexually Transmitted Infections

Infection	Common Symptoms	Treatment/Intervention/ Counseling
HIV	Acute HIV - Fever - Lymphadenopathy - Sore throat - Rash - Myalgia/arthralgia - Diarrhea - Weight loss - Headache - Mucocutaneous ulcers[11] - Can be asymptomatic Chronic HIV - Persistent generalized lymphadenopathy - Low-grade fever - Fatigue - Night sweats[9]	- Patients with symptoms of HIV or those who have been exposed to HIV should be seen by a healthcare provider. - Treatment for HIV includes a combination of antiretroviral medications. - Sexual partners should be offered postexposure prophylaxis with combination antiretrovirals.[2]
C. trachomatis (chlamydia)	- Cervicitis - Dysuria - Vaginal discharge - Menstrual irregularities *Can be asymptomatic.[4]	- Patients with symptoms of chlamydia or those who have been exposed to this infection should be seen by a healthcare provider. - First line treatments: azithromycin or doxycycline.

(continued)

TABLE 19.1 Common Symptoms of Sexually Transmitted Infections (*continued*)

Infection	Common Symptoms	Treatment/Intervention/ Counseling
		▪ Patients should abstain from sexual activity for 7 days following treatment and until 7 days after all sexual partners are treated. Recent sexual partners (sexual exposure was less than 60 days before onset of symptoms or diagnosis) and the most recent sexual partner should be referred for evaluation and treatment of chlamydia.[2]
N. gonorrhoeae (gonorrhea)	▪ Dysuria ▪ Vaginal discharge ▪ Vaginal bleeding between menstrual cycles *Can be asymptomatic.[5]	▪ Patients with symptoms of gonorrhea or those who have been exposed to this infection should be seen by a healthcare provider. ▪ First-line treatment is ceftriaxone plus azithromycin. Ceftriaxone and azithromycin should be administered on the same day. ▪ Patients with a gonorrhea infection should abstain from sexual activity for 7 days after treatment and until 7 days after all sexual partners are treated. ▪ Recent sexual partners (sexual exposure was less than 60 days before onset of symptoms or diagnosis) and the most recent sexual partner should be referred for evaluation and testing.[2]
Syphilis	Primary syphilis ▪ Ulcer or chancre Secondary syphilis ▪ Rash ▪ Mucocutaneous lesions ▪ Lymphadenopathy	▪ Patients with symptoms of syphilis should be seen by a healthcare provider. ▪ Patients who have had sexual contact in the last 90 days with someone with a diagnosis of syphilis should schedule an

(continued)

TABLE 19.1 Common Symptoms of Sexually Transmitted Infections (*continued*)

Infection	Common Symptoms	Treatment/Intervention/ Counseling
	Tertiary syphilis ▪ Gummatous lesions ▪ Cardiac lesions ▪ Tabes dorsalis ▪ General paresis Latent syphilis ▪ Asymptomatic[2]	appointment for syphilis treatment. Patients should be treated for syphilis even if serologic test results are negative. Serologic testing should be performed 6-12 months after treatment. First-line treatment: ▪ Penicillin G benzathine ▪ Duration of treatment depends on the suspected stage of syphilis, and therefore will be determined by the provider.
HSV	▪ Vesicles on or around the genitals, rectum, or mouth Initial outbreak ▪ Fever ▪ Body aches ▪ Swollen lymph nodes ▪ Headache Recurrent HSV outbreaks ▪ Genital pain ▪ Tingling pain in legs, hips, or buttocks ▪ Can be asymptomatic.[6]	▪ Patients with symptoms of HSV should be seen by a healthcare provider. ▪ Patient should abstain from sexual activity when herpes lesions are present or herpes symptoms are present. However, the virus can still be transmitted to sexual partners when HSV symptoms are present. ▪ Sexual partners of someone with herpes simplex virus should be advised to use condoms and be referred for testing to see if they are infected with HSV.[6] ▪ Sitz baths are helpful to relieve dysuria secondary to multiple ulcerations from HSV outbreak. Analgesic may also be necessary for women with multiple painful HSV ulcers.[10] Commonly prescribed medications: ▪ Acyclovir ▪ Famciclovir

(*continued*)

TABLE 19.1 Common Symptoms of Sexually Transmitted Infections (*continued*)

Infection	Common Symptoms	Treatment/Intervention/Counseling
		▪ Valacyclovir ▪ Antiviral therapy should be started within 72 hours of symptoms. Recurrent HSV outbreaks ▪ Episodic therapy involves patients starting therapy at first sign of prodromal symptoms of HSV outbreak.[10] ▪ Chronic suppressive therapy is also available for patients who have frequent and severe HSV outbreaks, or for people who wish to reduce the risk of transmission to uninfected sexual partner.
HPV	Anogenital warts ▪ Flat, popular, or pedunculated growths that can be painful or itchy Cervical cancer ▪ Abnormal pap smear and positive HPV testing Asymptomatic until advanced disease.[2]	Anogenital warts ▪ Patients with symptoms of anogenital warts should make an appointment with a healthcare provider. Patient applied treatment for anogenital warts includes: ▪ Imiquimod cream ▪ Podofilox solution or gel ▪ Sinecatechins 15% ointment. Provider administered treatment for anogenital warts includes: ▪ Cryotherapy ▪ Surgical removal ▪ Trichloroacetic acid ▪ Bichloroacetic acid ▪ Most anogenital warts respond to treatment within 3 months of therapy.

(*continued*)

TABLE 19.1 Common Symptoms of Sexually Transmitted Infections (*continued*)

Infection	Common Symptoms	Treatment/Intervention/Counseling
		■ It is recommended to avoid sexual contact with new partners until warts are gone. However, HPV might still be present and able to be transmitted to new partners. ■ HPV testing of sex partners of persons with genital warts is not recommended.[2]
Trichomonas vaginalis **(trichomoniasis)**	■ Malodorous, yellow-green vaginal discharge ■ Vulvar irritation ■ Urinary discomfort ■ Can be asymptomatic.[7]	■ Patients with symptoms of trichomoniasis or those who have been exposed to trichomoniasis should be seen by a healthcare provider. Commonly prescribed treatments: ■ Metronidazole ■ Tinidazole ■ Treatment of sexual partners is recommended. ■ It is recommended to avoid sexual contact until patient and all sexual partners are treated and symptoms have resolved. ■ Retesting should be 3 months after treatment.[2]
HBV	Acute hepatitis B infection ■ Fever ■ Fatigue ■ Anorexia ■ Nausea ■ Vomiting ■ Abdominal pain ■ Dark urine ■ Clay-colored bowel movements ■ Joint paint ■ Jaundice	■ Patients with symptoms of Hepatitis B should make appointment with a healthcare provider. ■ Sexual partners of someone with HBV infection should be tested and should receive the first dose of hepatitis B vaccine if not previously vaccinated. Acute hepatitis B infection ■ Treatment for acute hepatitis B infection is supportive care.

(*continued*)

TABLE 19.1 Common Symptoms of Sexually Transmitted Infections (*continued*)

Infection	Common Symptoms	Treatment/Intervention/Counseling
	Chronic hepatitis B Infection ▪ Asymptomatic[8]	▪ Person with HBV infection should be counseled to avoid or limit alcohol consumption, obtain vaccination about against hepatitis A, and avoid medications that can be toxic to the liver.[2] Chronic hepatitis B infection ▪ There are several antiviral medications available for the treatment of chronic HBV infection.[11]

HBV, Hepatitis B Virus; HPV, human papillomavirus; HSV, herpes simplex virus.i

➡ RED FLAGS

Pelvic pain: Pelvic inflammatory disease (PID) may present with pelvic pain in the lower abdomen, fever, vaginal discharge with foul order, pain, and/or bleeding when having sex, dysuria, or bleeding between menstrual cycles.[12] Prompt recognition and treatment is vital, as PID can lead to infertility. The nurse should alert a provider if the patient reports any potential symptoms, as an urgent clinic visit or ED visit might be necessary. PID is most commonly treated with ceftriaxone and a 14-day course of doxycycline, with or without metronidazole.[2] Parenteral treatment may be necessary in certain cases.

Neurological symptoms: Neurosyphilis signs may include headache, confusion, nausea, vomiting, stiff neck, or visual acuity impairment.[13] If neurosyphilis is suspected, the patient should be sent to the ED.

⊙ SPECIAL POPULATION CONSIDERATIONS

▪ **Pregnancy:** Pregnant women should have sexually transmitted disease (STD) screening for maternal and fetal well-being.

COMMONLY PRESCRIBED MEDICATIONS

TABLE 19.2 Commonly Prescribed Medications for Treatment of Sexually Transmitted Infections

Medicine	Common Side Effects	Common Interactions
Azithromycin[14]	Vomiting, diarrhea, nausea	Azithromycin may increase the serum concentration of ivermectin and vitamin K antagonists such as warfarin.
Doxycycline[15]	Diarrhea, nasopharyngitis, sinusitis, upper abdominal pain	Antacids, multivitamins, and bismuth subsalicylate may decrease the absorption of doxycycline. Doxycycline can diminish the therapeutic effect of penicillin. Doxycycline may enhance the anticoagulant effect of vitamin K antagonists such as warfarin. Doxycycline serum levels can be decreased if taken with high-fat meal or milk (15).
Ceftriaxone[16]	Induration at injection site, skin tightness, eosinophilia, thrombocytosis, diarrhea	Ceftriaxone may enhance the nephrotoxic effect of aminoglycosides and the anticoagulant effect of vitamin K antagonists such as warfarin.
Benzathine Penicillin G[17]	Hypotension, tachycardia, anxiety, dizziness, nausea, vomiting, inflammation at injection site, pain at injection site	Tetracyclines may diminish the effect of penicillin. Penicillin may enhance the anticoagulant effect of vitamin K antagonists such as warfarin.
Valacyclovir[18]	Headache, nausea, abdominal pain, increased serum AST, increased serum ALT, nasopharyngitis	Valacyclovir may diminish the effects of the varicella virus vaccine and zoster vaccine.
Acyclovir[19]	Malaise, headache, increased serum creatinine, nausea, vomiting, diarrhea, skin rash	Acyclovir may diminish the effects of the varicella virus vaccine and the zoster vaccine.

(continued)

TABLE 19.2 Commonly Prescribed Medications for Treatment of Sexually Transmitted Infections (*continued*)

Medicine	Common Side Effects	Common Interactions
Famciclovir[20]	Headache, nausea, diarrhea, vomiting, flatulence, dysmenorrhea, fatigue, neutropenia	Famciclovir may diminish the effects of the varicella virus vaccine and zoster vaccine
Podofilox 0.5% solution or gel[21]	Localized burning, local pain, skin erosion, local inflammation, headache, erythema, and local pruritus	No known significant drug interactions
Imiquimod 3.75% or 5% cream[22]	Localized erythema, xeroderma, crusted skin, sclerosis, localized vesiculation, localized edema, upper respiratory infection, headache, fatigue, sinusitis	Tacrolimus cream may enhance the toxic effect of imiquimod.
Sinecatechins[23]	Localized burning, local discomfort, erythema, pruritus, skin erosion, skin sclerosis, vesicular eruption, local pain, dermal ulcer, localized edema	There are no known significant interactions.
Metronidazole[24]	Headache, nausea, vaginitis, metallic taste, abdominal pain, diarrhea, flu-like symptoms	Metronidazole can enhance the toxic effect of alcohol and lithium. Disulfiram may enhance the toxic effects of metronidazole. Mebendazole and ritonavir may enhance the toxic effects of metronidazole. Metronidazole may increase the serum concentration of vitamin K antagonists.
Tinidazole[25]	Nausea, anorexia, dysgeusia, vulvovaginal candidiasis	Tinidazole may enhance the toxic effect of disulfiram. Tinidazole may diminish the therapeutic effect of lactobacillus and estriol

ALT, alanine transaminase; AST, aspartate aminotransferase.

MANAGING SIDE EFFECTS

Jarisch–Herxheimer reaction is an acute reaction that usually occurs with the first 24 hours after initiation of syphilis treatment. Symptoms include fever, headache, and myalgia. Antipyretics can be used to help manage symptoms.[2]

SUMMARY

- STIs are more common among the adolescent population.[2]
- Many STIs are asymptomatic.
- Routine screening is necessary in the adolescent population for some STIs to prevent transmission and health complications.
- Patients should always be encouraged to use condoms to help prevent transmission of STIs. It is also important to inform patients that hormonal contraceptive options do not protect again STIs.

RELATED PROTOCOLS

- **CDC STI treatment and testing guidelines**
- Expedited partner therapy (EPT)-treating sexual partner for STI without examination.[2] EPT is legal in most states for treatment of *C. trachomatis* and *N. gonorrhea*.
- HPV vaccination can reduce likelihood of acquiring HPV.[2]
- Hepatitis B vaccination can reduce likelihood of acquiring HBV.[2]
- Dontspreadit.org website: this is a website that allows for patients to anonymously notify their partner(s) about an STI.
- Chapters 22 and 23: Vulvovaginitis
- Chapter 13: Acute Pelvic Pain
- Chapter 14: Chronic Pelvic Pain

References

1. Ghanem KG, Tuddeneham S. Screening for sexually transmitted infections. In: Post TW, ed. *UpToDate*. Waltham, MA: UpToDate Inc. April 21, 2020. https://www.uptodate.com. Accessed July 26, 2020.
2. Workowski KA, Bolan GA. Sexually transmitted diseases treatment guidelines, 2015. Centers for Disease Control and Prevention. *MMWR Recomm Rep.* 2015;64(RR–03):1.
3. Centers for Disease Control. Chlamydia-CDC fact sheet. https://www.cdc.gov/std/chlamydia/stdfact-chlamydia.htm. Accessed June 22, 2019.
4. Stamm WE. Chlamydia trachomatis infections of the adult. In: Holmes KK, Sparling PF, Mardh PA, et al. eds. *Sexually Transmitted Diseases*. 4th ed. New York, NY: Mcgraw-Hill; 2008:575.
5. Centers for Disease Control. Gonorrhea-CDC fact sheet. https://www.cdc.gov/std/gonorrhea/stdfact-gonorrhea.htm. Accessed June 20, 2019.
6. Centers for Disease Control. Genital herpes-CDC fact sheet (detailed). https://www.cdc.gov/std/herpes/stdfact-herpes-detailed.htm. Accessed June 16, 2019.
7. Centers for Disease Control. Trichomoniasis-CDC fact sheet. https://www.cdc.gov/std/trichomonas/stdfact-trichomoniasis.htm. Accessed on June 23, 2019.
8. Centers for Disease Control. Hepatitis B questions and answers for health professionals. https://www.cdc.gov/hepatitis/hbv/hbvfaq.htm. Accessed June 15, 2019.

9. Osmond D, Chaisson R, Moss A, et al. Lymphadenopathy in asymptomatic patients seropositive for HIV. *N Engl J Med.* 1987;317:246.

10. Albrecht MA. Treatment of genital herpes simplex virus infection. In: Post TW, ed. *UpToDate.* Waltham, MA: UpToDate Inc; June 4, 2019. https://www.uptodate.com. Accessed June 22, 2019.

11. Terrault NA, Bzowej NH, Chang KM, Hwang JP, Jonas MM, Murad MH. AASLD guidelines for treatment of chronic hepatitis B. Hepatology. 2016;63(1):261–83.

12. Centers for Disease Control. Pelvic inflammatory disease (PID)-CDC fact sheet. https://www.cdc.gov/std/pid/stdfact-pid.htm. Accessed June 13, 2019.

13. Marra CM. Neurosyphillis. In: Post TW, ed. *UpToDate.* Waltham, MA: UpToDate Inc. December 21, 2018. https://www.uptodate.com. Accessed June 22, 2019.

14. Azithromycin. *Lexi-Drugs. Lexicomp.* Riverwoods, IL: Wolters Kluwer Health, Inc. http://online.lexi.com. Accessed June 18, 2019.

15. Doxycycline. *Lexi-Drugs. Lexicomp.* Riverwoods, IL: Wolters Kluwer Health, Inc. http://online.lexi.com. Accessed June 18, 2019.

16. Ceftriaxone. *Lexi-Drugs. Lexicomp.* Riverwoods, IL: Wolters Kluwer Health, Inc. http://online.lexi.com. Accessed June 18, 2019.

17. Benzathine Penicillin G. *Lexi-Drugs. Lexicomp.* Riverwoods, IL: Wolters Kluwer Health, Inc. http://online.lexi.com. Accessed June 18, 2019.

18. Valacyclovir. *Lexi-Drugs. Lexicomp.* Riverwoods, IL: Wolters Kluwer Health, Inc. http://online.lexi.com. Accessed June 18, 2019.

19. Acyclovir. *Lexi-Drugs. Lexicomp.* Riverwoods, IL: Wolters Kluwer Health, Inc. http://online.lexi.com. Accessed June 18, 2019.

20. Famiciclovir. *Lexi-Drugs. Lexicomp.* Riverwoods, IL: Wolters Kluwer Health, Inc. http://online.lexi.com. Accessed June 18, 2019.

21. Podofilox. *Lexi-Drugs. Lexicomp.* Riverwoods, IL: Wolters Kluwer Health, Inc. http://online.lexi.com. Accessed June 18, 2019.

22. Imiquimod. *Lexi-Drugs. Lexicomp.* Riverwoods, IL: Wolters Kluwer Health, Inc. http://online.lexi.com. Accessed June 18, 2019.

23. Sinecatechins. *Lexi-Drugs. Lexicomp.* Riverwoods, IL: Wolters Kluwer Health, Inc. http://online.lexi.com. Accessed June 18, 2019.

24. Metronidazole. *Lexi-Drugs. Lexicomp.* Riverwoods, IL: Wolters Kluwer Health, Inc. http://online.lexi.com. Accessed June 18, 2019.

25. Tinidazole. *Lexi-Drugs. Lexicomp.* Riverwoods, IL: Wolters Kluwer Health, Inc. http://online.lexi.com. Accessed June 18, 2019.

UNPROTECTED INTERCOURSE/ EMERGENCY CONTRACEPTION
Dana Lenobel

INTRODUCTION

Vaginal intercourse is considered to be unprotected anytime a male's penis enters a female's vagina without the use of a condom. Penetration may be shallow or deep and can include ejaculation. Patients often call the gynecology office with concerns regarding unprotected intercourse or regarding concerns for a broken condom during intercourse.

Unprotected intercourse occurs because of many different reasons. First, the patient may be using hormonal contraception or an intrauterine device (IUD). First, the patient and/or partner may not think it is possible to conceive or contract sexually transmitted infections (STIs) and thus may choose not to use a condom. Even if condoms are used, condoms are sometimes made with imperfections and can also break during intercourse, resulting in unwanted exposure. Second, drugs and alcohol may be involved during unprotected intercourse. Finally, a patient may have nonconsensual or coercive unprotected intercourse.

When a patient reports that they had unprotected intercourse, the nurse should assess whether the patient is using another form of contraception. If the patient is using a form of hormonal contraception, or has a copper IUD in place, the nurse should refer to Chapters 2 through 7 in this triage book addressing methods of contraception in order to determine if emergency contraception (EC) is needed. If the patient is not using an effective form of contraception or is not consistently using hormonal contraception correctly, establishing the timing for the unprotected intercourse event is important for determining what kind of EC is appropriate for the patient. The nurse should also assess if this unprotected intercourse was forced and if the patient feels safe.

It is important to determine whether the sexual activity was forced or coerced in any way and/or if any drugs or alcohol were used. Any forced intercourse within the pediatric and adolescent gynecology population must be reported based on state guidelines. Involving social work in this circumstance is also helpful. Specific reporting laws in each specific state can be found online through Child Welfare Information Gateway.[1] Only 10% to 15% of sexual assaults are reported to police, and females who know their assailant are less likely to report the assault.[2] Patients involved in forced or coercive intercourse should have an evaluation by a provider specifically trained to treat patients that were sexually assaulted.[1] Teenagers and young adults aged 12 to 34 years old have the highest rates of sexual assault.[1] Adolescents with disabilities are also at an increased risk of sexual assault. When the patient discloses she was sexually assaulted it is important to remain nonjudgmental.[1]

Unprotected intercourse can cause psychological effects, an unplanned pregnancy, or an STI. EC is an option to help prevent an unplanned pregnancy and can be used more than once in a menstrual cycle; however, if this is the case, a hormonal contraception method is the preferred approach.[3]

CLINICAL PEARL BOX 1

■ A routine pelvic exam, pregnancy test, and/or lab testing are NOT required prior to using oral emergency contraception (EC).[3,4] Unless a patient has missed her menses or thinks she may be pregnant, EC should not be delayed.[5]

COMMON PATIENT CONCERNS

■ Pregnancy risk
■ Contraction of a sexually transmitted infection
■ Selection of emergency contraceptive option
■ Vomiting following use of emergency contraceptive pills
■ Irregular bleeding following EC

⊙ KEY QUESTIONS TO ASK

■ When did the unprotected vaginal intercourse take place?
■ Was the unprotected intercourse consensual?
■ When was the patient's last menstrual cycle?
■ Does the patient feel safe?
■ Is the patient using any type of hormonal birth control? Is the patient using the hormone appropriately?
■ Is the patient having any pelvic pain, vaginal discharge, itching, or odor?
■ Is the patient having any abnormal vaginal bleeding?

TABLE 20.1 Patient Concerns and Symptoms Regarding Unprotected Vaginal Intercourse

Concerns/ Symptoms	Intervention/Delegation	Commonly Prescribed Medications
Pregnancy risk	▪ The risk depends on if they had intercourse in the fertile window, how many unprotected intercourse exposures she had within the cycle, and use of a hormonal contraceptive.[6] ▪ Patients with multiple episodes of unprotected intercourse in the cycle are at highest risk of conceiving. ▪ The nurse should collect enough information as possible for the provider to help decide if the patient is a candidate for EC. The dates of the patient's LMP and the dates of unprotected intercourse should be noted.	▪ EC ▪ Copper IUD
Exposure to an STI	▪ The patient should be told that anybody who has unprotected intercourse is at an increased risk for an STI, which includes gonorrhea, chlamydia, trichomonas, genital herpes, genital warts, HIV, Hepatitis B, Hepatitis C, syphilis. ▪ These patients should consider a pelvic exam with genital swabs and obtain sexually transmitted infection serology. ▪ Signs and symptoms of an STI should be discussed (refer to Chapter 19 on sexually transmitted infections). ▪ The nurse should offer an office visit for the patient to undergo screening for STIs. ▪ If the patient's partner has a known or suspected STI, the nurse should notify the provider for a sooner office visit, as earlier intervention may be recommended.	

(*continued*)

TABLE 20.1 Patient Concerns and Symptoms Regarding Unprotected Vaginal Intercourse (*continued*)

Concerns/ Symptoms	Intervention/Delegation	Commonly Prescribed Medications
Vomiting following oral EC	▨ The nurse should instruct the patient to repeat the dose if the vomiting occurred within 3 hours of ingestion.[7]	
Menstrual irregularities following EC	▨ EC users who do not have a menses within three weeks of taking the EC should take a pregnancy test.[8] ▨ The patient's period will generally restart within one week of anticipated menstrual date.[9] ▨ Irregular bleeding can also occur and persist for a month after taking oral EC.[3] ▨ If spotting or bleeding does not resolve a pregnancy test should be obtained. ▨ Of note, the use of the copper IUD should not impact the menstrual period given there are no hormones in the copper IUD.	

EC, emergency contraception; IUD, intrauterine device; LMP, last menstrual period; STI, sexually transmitted infection.

CLINICAL PEARL BOX 2

Initiating other contraceptive options following use of emergency contraception (EC):

▨ Ulipristal acetate (UPA): there should be a 5-day delay after taking UPA before initiating hormonal contraception due to drug interactions.[10]

▨ Levonorgestrel (LNG) oral: initiate the contraceptive method at the same time as LNG EC and abstain from intercourse or use a backup method for seven days.[5]

▨ Yuzpe method: can start any contraception method after taking the second dose of EC pill and abstain from intercourse or use a backup method for seven days.[5]

➡ RED FLAGS

■ **Safety concerns:** If the unprotected intercourse was not consensual and the patient is in immediate danger, the patient should hang up and call 9-1-1. If the patient is having thoughts of self-harm or suicide, it is important that the nurse identify the patient's current location and whether the patient has a plan. If the patient has a plan and is in immediate danger, the nurse should notify a guardian or someone in the home and contact the police.

(O) SPECIAL POPULATION CONSIDERATIONS

1. Breastfeeding: no restrictions on taking ulipristal acetate (UPA) or levonorgestrel (LNG) EC.[5]
2. Current pelvic inflammatory disease: should not use the copper IUD and oral EC should be considered.
3. Uterine anomaly: should not use the copper IUD.
4. Pregnancy: it is possible that a pregnancy existed before taking EC, the EC did not work properly, or a pregnancy resulted after EC was used. There are no known adverse effects of EC on pregnancy.[8] The risk of future fertility is not impacted if EC is used.[8]

COMMONLY PRESCRIBED MEDICINE

EC is any medication or product used to prevent pregnancy after unprotected intercourse. It must be initiated within a specific time frame in order to be effective. Emergency contraceptives work by disrupting the timing of ovulation or preventing fertilization of an ovulated egg.[10] It is important to note that EC is not a drug or method that is used to induce an abortion.[10] Any woman who had unprotected intercourse or under-protected intercourse (condom breaking) and wants to reduce their risk of pregnancy is a candidate for EC.[3] Pregnancy is the only absolute contraindication to oral EC and copper IUD.[11,12] A patient with a current pelvic inflammatory disease or uterine anomaly is a contraindication to the copper IUD.

The copper IUD is used as an EC method. Oral EC methods include UPA and LNG.

TABLE 20.2 Comparison of Copper IUD, Ulipristal Acetate, and Levonorgestrel

	Copper IUD	Ulipristal acetate 30 mg	Levonorgestrel 1.5 mg
Pregnancy risk	0.1%	Less than <2%	Less than <3%
Timing	The IUD should be placed up to 5 days after UPI, but may be effective at any time in the menstrual cycle if pregnancy is excluded.	Effective up to 5 days following UPI.	Effective up to 3 days after UPI, although may be effective up to 5 days.
When to initiate hormonal contraceptives following EC	Effective for contraception immediately after insertion.	Wait 5 days to begin hormonal contraceptive option.	May start contraception immediately.

EC, emergency contraception; IUD, intrauterine device; UPI, unprotected intercourse.

Source: From Cleland K, Zhu H, Goldstuck N, et al. The efficacy of intrauterine devices for emergency contraception: a systematic review of 35 years of experience. *Hum Reprod.* 2012;27:1994. doi:10.1093/humrep/des140; Glasier AF, Cameron ST, Fine PM, et al. Ulipristal acetate versus levonorgestrel for emergency contraception: a randomised non-inferiority trial and meta-analysis. *Lancet.* 2010;375:555. doi:10.1016/S0140-6736(10)60101-8; Shen J, Che Y, Showell E, et al. Interventions for emergency contraception. *Cochrane Database Syst Rev.* 2019;8:CD001324. doi:10.1002/14651858.CD001324.pub6; Turok DK, Godfrey EM, Wojdyla D, et al. Copper T380 intrauterine device for emergency contraception: highly effective at any time in the menstrual cycle. *Hum Reprod.* 2013;28:2672. doi:10.1093/humrep/det330; Emergency Contraceptive Pills: Medical and Service Delivery Guidance. International consortium for emergency contraception 2018. https://www.cecinfo.org/wp-content/uploads/2018/12/ICEC-guides_FINAL.pdf. Accessed on March 09, 2019; Noé G, Croxatto HB, Salvatierra AM, et al. Contraceptive efficacy of emergency contraception with levonorgestrel given before or after ovulation. *Contraception.* 2011;84:486. doi:10.1016/j.contraception.2011.03.006; Providing Ongoing Hormonal Contraception after Use of Emergency Contraceptive Pills. American society for emergency contraception 2016. http://americansocietyforec.org/uploads/3/4/5/6/34568220/asec_fact_sheet-_hormonal_contraception_after_ec.pdf. Accessed on March 09, 2019; Glasier A, Cameron ST, Blithe D, et al. Can we identify women at risk of pregnancy despite using emergency contraception? Data from randomized trials of ulipristal acetate and levonorgestrel. *Contraception.* 2011;84:363. doi:10.1016/j.contraception.2011.02.009.

MANAGING SIDE EFFECTS

Overall EC methods are safe and effective. Each method varies in its potential side effects. It is important to note that EC methods do not decrease the chances of getting an STI.

The copper IUD side effects can include abdominal or pelvic pain resulting from insertion, bleeding, uterine perforation, or infection.

Both UPA and LNG are exceptionally safe and avoid the rare major complications of combined hormonal contraception, specifically estrogen-related thrombogenic events. Common side effects of UPA include headache, abdominal pain, nausea, dysmenorrhea, fatigue, and dizziness.[11] Common side effects of LNG include menstrual changes, nausea, lower abdominal pain, fatigue, headache, dizziness, breast pain, and vomiting.[12]

SUMMARY

- Unprotected vaginal intercourse is anytime a male's penis enters a female's vagina without the use of a condom.
- The time when the unprotected intercourse took place is important to help determine which kind of EC may be appropriate for the patient.
- The nurse should also assess if this unprotected intercourse was forced and if the patient feels safe.

RELATED PROTOCOLS

- Reporting laws in each specific state can be found online through Child Welfare Information Gateway.[1] This website will give information on each state and when and to who a provider should report nonconsensual intercourse. The age of consent to intercourse varies from state to state. It may be mandatory to report that intercourse occurred even if it was consensual.
- The nurse should be familiar with their specific facility's policy if a patient was sexually assaulted and specific referring centers in the area.
- The nurse should also familiarize themselves with their facility's policy in case a patient endorses suicidal thoughts or safety concerns related to the unprotected intercourse.

References

1. Crawford-Jakubiak JE, Alderman EM, Leventhal JM, et al. Care of the adolescent after an acute sexual assault. *Pediatrics*. 2017;139. doi:10.1542/peds
2. Jones JS, Alexander C, Wynn BN, et al. Why women don't report sexual assault to the police: the influence of psychosocial variables and traumatic injury. *J Emerg Med*. 2009;36:417. doi:10.1016/j.jemermed.2007.10.077
3. The American College of Obstetricians and Gynecologists. Practice bulletin No. 152: Emergency contraception. *Obstet Gynecol*. 2015; 126:e1. Reaffirmed 2018. doi:10.1097/AOG.0000000000001047
4. *FSRH Guideline Emergency Contraception*. UK: Faculty of Sexual & Reproductive Healthcare; December 2017.
5. CEU Clinical Guidance: Emergency Contraception - December 2017. Faculty of reproductive and sexual healthcare of the royal college of obstetricians and Gynaecologists. www.fsrh.org/standards-and-guidance/current-clinical-guidance/emergency-contraception/. Accessed on March 27, 2019.
6. Espinós JJ, Rodríguez-Espinosa J, Senosiain R, et al. The role of matching menstrual data with hormonal measurements in evaluating effectiveness

of postcoital contraception. *Contraception.* 1999;60:243. doi:10.1016/S0010-7824(99)00090-6

7. Curtis KM, Tepper NK, Jatlaoui TC, et al. U.S. Medical eligibility criteria for contraceptive use, 2016. *MMWR Recomm Rep.* 2016;65:1. doi:10.15585/mmwr.rr6503a1

8. Trussell J, Cleland K, Bimla Schwarz E. Emergency contraception. In: Hatcher RA, Nelson AL, Trussell J, et al., eds. *Contraceptive Technology, 21.* New York, NY: Ayer Company Publishers, Inc.; 2018:329-365.

9. Randomised controlled trial of levonorgestrel versus the Yuzpe regimen of combined oral contraceptives for emergency contraception. Task force on postovulatory methods of fertility regulation. *Lancet.* 1998;352:428. doi:10.1016/S0140-6736(98)05145-9

10. Turok, D. Emergency contraception. *UpToDate.* https://www.uptodate.com/contents/emergency-contraception?search=emergency%20contraception&source=search_result&selectedTitle=1~150&usage_type=default&display_rank=1. Accessed on March 22, 2019.

11. Ulipristal acetate. US FDA approved product information. National library of medicine. www.dailymed.nlm.nih.gov/dailymed/. Accessed on March 22, 2019.

12. Plan B (levonorgestrel). *US FDA Prescribing Information.* North Wales, PA: Teva Women's Health, Inc.; September, 2017. https://www.accessdata.fda.gov/drugsatfda_docs/label/2017/021045s016lbl.pdf. Accessed March 9, 2019.

13. Cleland K, Zhu H, Goldstuck N, et al. The efficacy of intrauterine devices for emergency contraception: a systematic review of 35 years of experience. *Hum Reprod.* 2012;27:1994. doi:10.1093/humrep/des140

14. Glasier AF, Cameron ST, Fine PM, et al. Ulipristal acetate versus levonorgestrel for emergency contraception: a randomised non-inferiority trial and meta-analysis. *Lancet.* 2010;375:555. doi:10.1016/S0140-6736(10)60101-8.

15. Shen J, Che Y, Showell E, et al. Interventions for emergency contraception. *Cochrane Database Syst Rev.* 2019;8:CD001324. doi:10.1002/14651858.CD001324.pub6

16. Turok DK, Godfrey EM, Wojdyla D, et al. Copper T380 intrauterine device for emergency contraception: highly effective at any time in the menstrual cycle. *Hum Reprod.* 2013;28:2672. doi:10.1093/humrep/det330

17. Emergency Contraceptive Pills: Medical and Service Delivery Guidance. International consortium for emergency contraception 2018. https://www.cecinfo.org/wp-content/uploads/2018/12/ICEC-guides_FINAL.pdf. Accessed on March 09, 2019.

18. Noé G, Croxatto HB, Salvatierra AM, et al. Contraceptive efficacy of emergency contraception with levonorgestrel given before or after ovulation. *Contraception.* 2011;84:486. doi:10.1016/j.contraception.2011.03.006

19. Providing Ongoing Hormonal Contraception after Use of Emergency Contraceptive Pills. American society for emergency contraception 2016. http://americansocietyforec.org/uploads/3/4/5/6/34568220/asec_fact_sheet-_hormonal_contraception_after_ec.pdf. Accessed on March 09, 2019.

20. Glasier A, Cameron ST, Blithe D, et al. Can we identify women at risk of pregnancy despite using emergency contraception? Data from randomized trials of ulipristal acetate and levonorgestrel. *Contraception.* 2011;84:363. doi:10.1016/j.contraception.2011.02.009

URINARY CONCERNS
Jessica Ginn

INTRODUCTION

There are many common urinary concerns in female children and adolescents, such as dysuria, urinary frequency, hematuria, urinary incontinence, and polyuria. These complaints can be self-limiting, signs of infection, or even life-threatening. Clinical evaluation is often warranted for urinary complaints so patients should be encouraged to make an appointment with a healthcare provider for most urinary concerns. The patient should be advised to go to the ED if she has symptoms of pelvic inflammatory disease (PID), pyelonephritis, or diabetic ketoacidosis (DKA).

CLINICAL PEARL BOX

If a patient is treated with an antibiotic, urinary symptoms should improve within 48 hours of initiating therapy.

COMMON PATIENT CONCERNS

- Dysuria (burning with urination)
- Hematuria (blood in the urine)
- Increased frequency or polyuria (increased urine amount)
- Dysuria associated with vaginal symptoms
- Lower abdominal pain
- Back pain
- Urinary incontinence
- Urinary incontinence with urinary urgency

⊙ KEY QUESTIONS TO ASK

- Is the patient experiencing any dysuria, urinary frequency, hematuria, or urinary incontinence?
- Does the patient have any associated fevers, back pain, abdominal pain, nausea, or vomiting?
- When did the patient first notice the symptoms?
- Is there any possibility of pregnancy?
- Is the patient sexually active?
- Is there an associated vaginal discharge?
- Does the patient ever experience polyuria, polydipsia, or polyphagia?
- Is the urine discolored?
- Does the patient have any chronic health conditions?
- Does the patient have constipation?

SYMPTOMS

TABLE 21.1 Acute Symptoms of Urinary Conditions

Acute Symptoms	Intervention/Delegation/ Counseling	Commonly Prescribed Medications
Dysuria	▪ This can be a sign of an uncomplicated lower UTI. Other common symptoms can include: urinary frequency, suprapubic pain, and hematuria.[2] ▪ The nurse should encourage the patient to drink more water, and take OTC pain medication until they can be seen in clinic for evaluation. ▪ Pyridium (can be purchased OTC)	▪ Nitrofurantoin[3] ▪ Trimethoprim-sulfamethoxazole[3] ▪ Fosfomycin[3] ▪ Pivmecillinam[3] ▪ Amoxicillin-Clavunate[4] ▪ Symptoms should improve within 48 hours of starting antibiotic.[1]
Dysuria associated with vaginal symptoms	▪ Dysuria with vaginal symptoms is less likely caused by a UTI and may be a sign of an STI.[6] ▪ Any type of vaginal symptom, including **discharge, irregular bleeding, vaginal itching, or discomfort**, can be a sign of an STI, such as chlamydia (*Chlamydia trachomatis*), gonorrhea (*Neisseria gonorrhoeae*), or trichomoniasis (*Trichomonas vaginalis*) infection.[6]	▪ Azithromycin or doxycycline[6] ▪ Ceftriaxone plus azithromycin. (ceftriaxone and azithromycin should be administered on the same day when using together).[6] ▪ Tinidazole or metronidazole[6] ▪ Abstinence is recommended for 7 days after treatment.

(continued)

TABLE 21.1 Acute Symptoms of Urinary Conditions (*continued*)

Acute Symptoms	Intervention/Delegation/Counseling	Commonly Prescribed Medications
	▪ The nurse should inquire if the patient is sexually active, and recommend the patient schedule an office visit for evaluation. ▪ Recommend abstaining from sexual activity until seen by healthcare provider.	▪ Recommend a test of cure visit for the patient in 3 months.[6]
Hematuria	▪ Blood in the urine can be a sign of a UTI.[2] ▪ This can also be a sign of a urinary stone. Other common symptoms of a urinary stone may include dysuria and flank pain.[8] ▪ The patient should be seen in clinic for a prompt evaluation if stable. ▪ If the associated pain is severe, the nurse should instruct the patient to go to the ED. ▪ Recommend supportive care, including hydration and OTC pain medication if needed.[12]	▪ Most patients with urinary stones can be managed with pain medication and increased fluid intake.[12]
Increased frequency or polyuria	▪ Increased frequency of urination can be a sign of a UTI, especially if associated with dysuria or other symptoms.[2] ▪ Increased frequency of urination can be a sign of pregnancy. If the patient is sexually active, the nurse should inquire about the patient's LMP and if any unprotected intercourse has occurred. If there is a chance of pregnancy, the nurse should recommend a UPT. ▪ If associated with **polydipsia** (increased thirst) or **polyphagia** (increased appetite), and/or weight loss, an evaluation for diabetes may be warranted.[9] The nurse should schedule a same-day clinic visit or recommend a same-day primary care office visit for further evaluation.	▪ Nitrofurantoin[3] ▪ Trimethoprim-sulfamethoxazole[3] ▪ Fosfomycin[3] ▪ Pivmecillinam[3] ▪ Amoxicillin-Clavunate[4] ▪ Symptoms should improve within 48 hours of starting antibiotic.[1]

(*continued*)

TABLE 21.1 Acute Symptoms of Urinary Conditions (*continued*)

Acute Symptoms	Intervention/Delegation/Counseling	Commonly Prescribed Medications
Lower abdominal pain	■ Lower abdominal pain can be a sign of a UTI. Other associated symptoms can include **dysuria, urinary frequency, and hematuria.**[2] Lower abdominal pain associated with **fever, vaginal discharge, pain associated with intercourse, and/or dysuria** can be a sign of pelvic inflammatory disease.[10] The patient should be seen in clinic for an urgent evaluation or sent to the ED if a clinic visit is not a possibility.	■ Ceftriaxone 250 mg intramuscular in a single dose and doxycycline[10] ■ Severe PID or Tubo-ovarian abscess may warrant admission to the hospital for IV antibiotics.[10]
Back pain	■ Back pain or tenderness can be a sign of pyelonephritis. Other common symptoms may include dysuria, hematuria, urinary frequency, plus **fever, chills, flank pain, nausea and/or vomiting.**[11] ■ If pyelonephritis is suspected, the patient should always be sent to the ED for immediate evaluation.	■ Different antibiotics are used based on severity of symptoms and if the patient is receiving treatment inpatient or outpatient.[5]

IM, intramuscular; IV, intravenous; LMP, last menstrual period; OTC, over the counter; PID, pelvic inflammatory disease; STI, sexually transmitted infection; TOA, Tubo-ovarian abscess; UPT, urine pregnancy test; UTI, urinary tract infection.

TABLE 21.2 Chronic Symptoms of Urinary Conditions

Chronic Symptoms	Intervention/Delegation/Counseling	Commonly Prescribed Medications
Urinary incontinence	■ This can be a sign of vaginal voiding. Vaginal voiding occurs when urine flows into the vagina following voiding. It occurs most commonly in patients with obesity, labial adhesions, and/or those who void with their legs closed.[14] ■ Recommend the patient sit backward on toilet while voiding and manually spread labia majora	None

(*continued*)

TABLE 21.2 Chronic Symptoms of Urinary Conditions (*continued*)

Chronic Symptoms	Intervention/Delegation/ Counseling	Commonly Prescribed Medications
	before voiding. The patient can also use a wide abduction of legs and a forward-leaning posture while voiding to help with vaginal voiding.[15]	
Urinary incontinence with urinary urgency	▪ This can be a sign of overactive bladder.[16] Urinary frequency may be another symptom present. ▪ Recommend reducing consumption of alcohol, caffeinated beverages, and carbonated beverages. Recommend consuming small amounts of liquid throughout the day, weight loss, avoiding smoking, pelvic floor exercises, and reducing constipation with high-iron diet. ▪ Urinalysis and urine culture to rule out urinary tract infection.	▪ None are approved by FDA. ▪ Oxybutinin ▪ Tolterodine ▪ This should always be managed by a urology provider or urogynecologist.

FDA, Food and Drug Administration; UA, urinalysis.

➡ RED FLAGS

Pyelonephritis: Symptoms may include dysuria, urinary frequency, suprapubic pain, and hematuria (signs of simple lower urinary tract infection) accompanied by fever, chills, flank pain, costovertebral angle tenderness (CVA) tenderness, nausea, and vomiting.[3] Patients with suspected pyelonephritis should always be sent to the ED.

PID: Common symptoms include dysuria, pain in lower abdomen, fever, vaginal discharge with foul order, pain, and/or bleeding when having sex, dysuria, or bleeding between menstrual cycles.[10] The patient should be seen in clinic for an urgent evaluation, or sent to the ED if a clinic visit is not a possibility.

DKA: Symptoms include polyuria, polydipsia, and polyphagia.[13] Patients with suspected DKA should be sent to the ED.

SPECIAL POPULATION CONSIDERATIONS

TABLE 21.3 Special Population Considerations for Urinary Conditions

Chronic Condition	Significance	Intervention/Delegation
Urologic abnormalities and renal abnormalities	More at risk for urinary tract infections and pyelonephritis.[17]	Encourage the patient to make an appointment with their healthcare provider as soon as possible. Instruct patient to go to ED if signs of pyelonephritis.
Immunosuppressed patients	More at risk for any type of infection.	Encourage patient to make an appointment with their healthcare provider as soon as possible. Instruct patient to go to ED if signs of systemic infection.

COMMONLY PRESCRIBED MEDICATIONS

TABLE 21.4 Commonly Prescribed Medications for Treatment of Urinary Conditions

Medicine	Common Side Effects	Common Interactions
Nitrofurantoin[18]	Headache, nausea, flatulence	Serum concentrations of nitrofurantoin are higher if taken with food. Nitrofurantoin may enhance the toxic effect of prilocaine and sodium nitrite.
Trimethoprim-sulfamethoxazole[19]	Skin rash, pruritus, abdominal pain, diarrhea, anorexia, nausea	Trimethoprim-sulfamethoxazole may increase the serum concentration of metformin. May increase the hyperkalemic effect of spironolactone. May enhance the anticoagulant effect of vitamin K antagonists[21]
Fosfomycin[20]	Diarrhea, nausea, abdominal pain, headache, vaginitis, rhinitis	May diminish the therapeutic effect of sodium picosulfate, lactobacillus, and estriol.
Pivmecillinam[21]	Diarrhea, nausea, vulvovaginal candidiasis	May increase serum concentration of methotrexate. May increase the anticoagulant effect of vitamin K antagonists. Tetracycline may diminish therapeutic effect of pivmecillinam.

(*continued*)

TABLE 21.4 Commonly Prescribed Medications for Treatment of Urinary Conditions (*continued*)

Medicine	Common Side Effects	Common Interactions
Azithromycin[22]	Vomiting, diarrhea, nausea	Azithromycin may increase the serum concentration of ivermectin and vitamin K antagonists such as warfarin.
Doxycycline[23]	Diarrhea, nasopharyngitis, sinusitis, upper abdominal pain, photosensitivity (sun sensitivity)	Antacids, multivitamins, and bismuth subsalicylate may decrease the absorption of doxycycline. Doxycycline can diminish the therapeutic effect of penicillin. Doxycycline may enhance the anticoagulant effect of vitamin K antagonists such as warfarin. Doxycycline serum levels can be decreased if taken with high-fat meal or milk.
Ceftriaxone[24]	Induration at injection site, skin tightness, eosinophilia, thrombocythemia, diarrhea	Ceftriaxone may enhance the nephrotoxic effect of aminoglycosides and the anticoagulant effect of vitamin K antagonists such as warfarin.
Tinidazole[25]	Nausea, anorexia, dysgeusia, vulvovaginal candidiasis	Tinidazole may enhance the toxic effect of disulfiram. It may diminish the therapeutic effect of lactobacillus and estriol.
Metronidazole[26]	Headache, nausea, vaginitis, metallic taste, abdominal pain, diarrhea, flu-like symptoms	Metronidazole can enhance the toxic effect of alcohol and lithium. Disulfiram may enhance the toxic effects of metronidazole. Mebendazole and ritonavir may enhance the toxic effects of metronidazole. Metronidazole may increase the serum concentration of vitamin K antagonists.

MANAGING SIDE EFFECTS

Do not take over the counter urinary tract infection pain reliever medication such as Phenazopyridine unless instructed by your healthcare provider. This may affect the results of a urine culture which could delay appropriate treatment.

SUMMARY

■ Urinary complaints are very common in female children and adolescents.

■ Urinary complaints can be a sign of many different conditions and most urinary complaints warrant a visit with a healthcare provider.

■ It is important for nursing staff to be able to identify urinary symptoms that can be signs of life-threatening conditions.

RELATED PROTOCOLS

■ Chapter 22: Pediatric Vulvovaginitis

■ Chapter 23: Adolescent Vulvovaginitis and Vaginal Discharge

References

1. Bachur R. Nonresponders: prolonged fever among infants with urinary tract infections. *Pediatrics*. 2000;105(5):E59. doi:10.1542/peds.105.5.e59
2. Bent S, Nallamothu, BK, Simel DL, et al. Does this woman have an acute uncomplicated urinary tract infection? *JAMA*. 2002;287:2701. doi:10.1001/jama.287.20.2701
3. Gupta K, Hooton TM. Acute cystitis in women: Post TW, ed. *UpToDate*. Waltham, MA: UpToDate Inc. https://www.uptodate.com. Accessed on June 22, 2020.
4. Shaikh N. Hoberman A. Urinary tract infections in infants older than one month and young children: Acute management, imaging, and prognosis: Post TW, ed. *UpToDate*. Waltham, MA: UpToDate Inc. https://www.uptodate.com. Accessed on July 27, 2020.
5. Gupta K, Hooton TM, Naber KG, et al. International clinical practice guidelines for the treatment of acute uncomplicated cystitis and pyelonephritis in women: a 2010 update by the infectious diseases society of America and the European society for microbiology and infectious diseases. *Clin Infect Dis*. 2011;52(5):e103. doi:10.1093/cid/ciq257
6. Workowski KA, Bolan GA. Sexually transmitted diseases treatment guidelines, 2015. Centers for Disease Control and Prevention. *MMWR Recomm Rep*. 2015; 64(RR-03):1.
7. Elton TJ, Roth CS, Berquist TH, Silverstein MD. A clinical prediction rule for the diagnosis of ureteral calculi in emergency departments. *J Gen Intern Med*. 1993;8(2):57. doi:10.1007/BF02599984
8. Curhan GC, Aronson MD, Preminger GM. Diagnosis and acute management of suspected nephrolithiasis in adults. In: Post TW, ed. *UpToDate*. Waltham, MA: UpToDate Inc. https://www.uptodate.com. Accessed on June 20, 2019.
9. Haller MJ, Atkinson MA, Schatz D. Type 1 diabetes mellitus: etiology, presentation, and management. *Pediatr Clin North Am*. 2005;52(6):1553. doi:10.1016/j.pcl.2005.07.006
10. Centers for Disease Control. Pelvic inflammatory disease (PID)-CDC Fact Sheet. https://www.cdc.gov/std/pid/stdfact-pid.htm. Accessed on June 13, 2019.
11. Fairley KF, Carson NE, Gutch RC, et al. Site of infection in acute urinary-tract infection in general practice. *Lancet*. 1971;2:615. doi:10.1016/S0140-6736(71)80066-1.

12. Springhart WP, Marguet CG, Sur RL, et al. Forced versus minimal intravenous hydration in management of acute renal colic: a randomized trial. *J Endourol.* 2006:20:713. doi:10.1089/end.2006.20.713

13. Glaser N. Clinical features and diagnosis of diabetic ketoacidosis in children and adolescents. In: Post TW, ed. *UpToDate.* Waltham, MA: UpToDate Inc. https://www.uptodate.com. Accessed on June 20, 2019.

14. Bernasconi M, Borsari A, Garzoni L, et al. Vaginal voiding: a common cause of daytime urinary leakage in girls. *J Pediatr Adolesc Gynecol.* 2009;22:347. doi:10.1016/j.jpag.2008.07.017

15. Nepple MD, Cooper CS. Etiology and clinical features of bladder dysfunction in children. In: Post TW, ed. *UpToDate.* Waltham, MA: UpToDate Inc. https://www.uptodate.com. Accessed on June 20, 2019.

16. Austin, PF, Bauer SB, Bower W, et al. The standardization of terminology of lower urinary tract function in children and adolescents; update report from the standardization committee of the international children's continence society. *J. Urol.* 2014;191:1863. doi:10.1016/j.juro.2014.01.110

17. Shaikh N, Hoberman A. Urinary tract infections in children; Epidemiology and risk factors. In: Post TW, ed. *UpToDate.* Waltham, MA: UpToDate Inc. https://www.uptodate.com. Accessed on June 20, 2019.

18. Nitrofurantoin. *Lexi-Drugs. Lexicomp.* Riverwoods, IL: Wolters Kluwer Health, Inc. http://online.lexi.com. Accessed June 18, 2019.

19. Trimethoprim-sulfamethoxazole. *Lexi-Drugs. Lexicomp.* Riverwoods, IL: Wolters Kluwer Health, Inc. http://online.lexi.com. Accessed June 18, 2019.

20. Fosfomycin. *Lexi-Drugs. Lexicomp.* Riverwoods, IL: Wolters Kluwer Health, Inc. http://online.lexi.com. Accessed June 18, 2019.

21. Pivmecillinam. *Lexi-Drugs. Lexicomp.* Riverwoods, IL: Wolters Kluwer Health, Inc. http://online.lexi.com. Accessed June 18, 2019.

22. Azithromycin. *Lexi-Drugs. Lexicomp.* Riverwoods, IL: Wolters Kluwer Health, Inc. http://online.lexi.com. Accessed June 18, 2019.

23. Doxycycline. *Lexi-Drugs. Lexicomp.* Riverwoods, IL: Wolters Kluwer Health, Inc. http://online.lexi.com. Accessed June 18, 2019.

24. Ceftriaxone. *Lexi-Drugs. Lexicomp.* Riverwoods, IL: Wolters Kluwer Health, Inc. http://online.lexi.com. Accessed June 18, 2019.

25. Tinidazole. *Lexi-Drugs. Lexicomp.* Riverwoods, IL: Wolters Kluwer Health, Inc. http://online.lexi.com. Accessed June 18, 2019.

26. Metronidazole. *Lexi-Drugs. Lexicomp.* Riverwoods, IL: Wolters Kluwer Health, Inc. http://online.lexi.com. Accessed June 18, 2019.

22

PEDIATRIC VULVOVAGINITIS

Jeanette Higgins

INTRODUCTION

Vulvitis is defined by is itching, burning, redness, or rash on the external genitalia. Vaginitis is the irritation of the vagina, and symptoms can include discharge and/or bleeding. When vaginitis and vulvitis occur together, it is called vulvovaginitis.

In this chapter, only prepubertal girls will be discussed. Adolescent vulvovaginitis will be discussed in Chapter 23.

Vulvovaginitis accounts for about 62% of pediatric gynecological problems in primary care.[1] The pediatric population is at higher risk for vulvovaginitis for a variety of reasons, including lack of vaginal estrogen, the smaller size of the labia minor and majora, an alkaline pH of the vagina, poor perineal hygiene, and the proximity of the urethra and anus to the vagina.[2] Up to 75% of vulvovaginitis cases in this population have a nonspecific cause and may resolve with improved vulvar hygiene and reassurance.[2]

CLINICAL PEARL BOX

HYGIENE TIPS[3,4]
- Wear cotton undergarments.
- Wear loose-fitting clothing.
- Wear nightgowns to bed instead of pants or pull-up sleepers.
- Avoid scented laundry detergents and avoid fabric softeners for undergarments.
- Wipe front to back after voiding or bowel movements (BMs).
- Wash hands frequently and thoroughly.
- Void with legs apart to prevent vaginal voiding.

DAILY BATHING TIPS[3]
- Encourage daily bathing.
- Avoid bubble baths and bath bombs.
- Avoid scented soaps.
- Soak in clean water prior to using soaps.
- Use soaps last before getting out of the bath.
- Rinse the genital area well.
- Pat the area dry or use a hairdryer on a cool setting to help dry the area.

Another cause may include sexually transmitted infections (STIs), which always warrants an emergent evaluation in a pediatric patient. Pinworms may also occur in this younger population and cause an array of both vaginal and rectal symptoms. Finally, there may be an underlying dermatologic condition such as lichen sclerosus and labial adhesions.

Treatment for vulvovaginitis depends on the underlying cause.[4] If there is an organism that is identified by culture, this would guide specific antibiotic treatment. If there is no identified organism, then antibiotics are not typically used as hygiene measures alone may result in resolution.

⊙ KEY QUESTIONS TO ASK

Vaginal itching
- When did the itching start?
- Is the itching worse at night?
- Are there any associated symptoms such as skin changes or discharge?
- Has the patient used any new soaps or laundry detergents?

Vaginal pain
- When did the pain start?
- How often does the pain occur? Daily, weekly?
- How long does the pain last?
- Is the pain a stabbing pain or more like an ache?
- Where is the pain? Can she point to where the pain occurs?

Bleeding
- Has menarche occurred?
- When did the bleeding start?
- How often does the bleeding occur?
- How much bleeding is occurring?
- Is there a chance there could be a foreign body?
- Is there a history of sexual abuse or trauma?
- Does the patient have a history of constipation? When was the last bowel movement? Are the stools hard or hard to push out? Is the patient taking any medications for the constipation?

Labial adhesions
- Has the patient been evaluated by the primary care physician?
- What creams or ointments have been used?
- How long have the creams or ointments been used?
- Did the creams or ointments help?

- Have the adhesions ever resolved?
- Have the adhesions ever been manually separated in the office or in the operating room?

Rash

- Is the patient in diapers during the day or night?
- What symptoms is the patient having? Is there any itching, dysuria, or redness?
- Is there any discharge? If so, what color is it? Does it have an odor?
- What medications, creams, or treatments have been tried? Did it help?
- Are there any irritant exposures, like soaps, detergents, bubble baths, and powders?
- Any recent infections in the family?

TABLE 22.1 Acute Symptoms of Pediatric Vulvovaginitis

Common Patient Concerns/ Symptoms	Counseling/Interventions	Medications Prescribed
Vaginal itching	- Patients with vaginal itching should have their skin examined by a parent or guardian. - Parents/guardians should look for redness, rash, lesions, bleeding, and/or discharge. - Tight-fitting clothing and non-cotton underwear can trigger symptoms of vulvovaginitis. Contact with harsh soaps, bubble baths, and laundry detergent may also result in irritation.[3] - The nurse should recommend avoiding any potential contact irritants. - An office visit for additional evaluation is recommended.	- Petroleum jelly - Fragrance-free barrier creams
Vaginal pain	- Vaginal pain is often hard for little kids to describe, so the nurse should have the parent ask the child to point to where the pain occurs. - Have the parent/guardian keep a pain/symptom diary. - The nurse should inquire about sexual abuse. If abuse is suspected, see "red flags."	- Petroleum jelly - Fragrance-free barrier creams

(*continued*)

TABLE 22.1 Acute Symptoms of Pediatric Vulvovaginitis (*continued*)

Common Patient Concerns/ Symptoms	Counseling/Interventions	Medications Prescribed
	▪ If any vaginal trauma is suspected, see "red flags." ▪ The nurse should recommend cool compresses to help relieve discomfort.	
Vaginal discharge	▪ Parents/guardians should note the color of discharge, how often it occurs, and any odor. These details should be recorded in a diary and brought to the appointment. ▪ Vaginal discharge that has an odor, associated bleeding, or yellow/green appearance needs to be evaluated urgently in the office. ▪ The nurse should inquire about potential introduction of a foreign body into the area, such as a small toy. ▪ All patients with vaginal discharge should be evaluated in clinic.	▪ Petroleum jelly ▪ Fragrance-free barrier creams
Vaginal bleeding	▪ Parent/guardians should note how often the bleeding is occurring, what color is the bleeding (bright red, dark brown), and when the bleeding started. ▪ The patient should be sent to the ED for any heavy vaginal bleeding and/or vaginal trauma such as a straddle injury. ▪ The nurse should inquire about sexual abuse. If abuse is suspected, the patient should be referred to the ED for immediate evaluation. ▪ These patients need an appointment for a visit.	▪ Petroleum jelly ▪ Fragrance-free barrier creams
Labial adhesions	▪ The nurse should inquire about any associated symptoms occurring from the adhesions, such as vaginal discomfort, difficulty with urination, and/or recurrent vaginal or urine infections. ▪ A provider should evaluate the patient in clinic.	▪ Topical steroid creams ▪ Topical estrogen therapy

(*continued*)

TABLE 22.1 Acute Symptoms of Pediatric Vulvovaginitis (*continued*)

Common Patient Concerns/ Symptoms	Counseling/Interventions	Medications Prescribed
	▪ Asymptomatic adhesions may not require treatment. ▪ Adhesions causing symptoms will likely need treatment.[5]	

TABLE 22.2 Chronic Symptoms of Pediatric Vulvovaginitis

Common Patient Concerns/ Symptoms	Counseling/Interventions	Medications Prescribed
Vaginal bleeding	▪ The patient should be sent to the ED for any heavy vaginal bleeding. ▪ The nurse should inquire about sexual abuse. If abuse is suspected, the patient should be referred to the ED for immediate evaluation. ▪ The nurse should inquire on pattern of the bleeding and any changes in bleeding since the previous office visit. ▪ These patients need an appointment for a visit.	▪ Petroleum jelly ▪ Fragrance-free barrier creams
Vaginal discharge	▪ Discharge that is yellow/green, blood tinged, and/or malodorous increases the likelihood of a foreign body in the vagina, such as a small toy or toilet paper. Anyone with a suspected foreign body needs to be seen urgently. ▪ Other causes include STIs. Should this concern arise, recommendations for prompt evaluation for sexual abuse should be advised.	▪ Antibiotics may be prescribed.
Vaginal itching	▪ The nurse should reinforce appropriate hygiene measures. ▪ The nurse should assess which contact irritants the patient has been avoiding, and help identify any additional triggers. ▪ For patients with known or suspected lichen sclerosis, the nurse should inquire on which	▪ Barrier creams ▪ Nystatin creams ▪ Albendazole, mebendazole, and/or pyrantel pamoate may be used for patients with pinworms.

(*continued*)

TABLE 22.2 Chronic Symptoms of Pediatric Vulvovaginitis (*continued*)

Common Patient Concerns/ Symptoms	Counseling/Interventions	Medications Prescribed
	treatment the patient is using, duration of treatment, and any response to treatment.	
	▪ If a patient was recently treated for pinworms and does not notice an improvement in symptoms, additional treatment may be warranted.[6] Family members may also need to be evaluated and treated for pinworms.	
	▪ Patients who do not notice an improvement in vaginal itching despite avoiding contact irritants and using recommended treatment should be reevaluated in clinic.	
Vaginal pain	▪ Ask the parent/guardian to keep a diary of pain, along with duration and resolution.	▪ Petroleum jelly ▪ Fragrance-free Barrier creams
	▪ The nurse should inquire about sexual abuse. If abuse is suspected, the patient should be referred to the ED for immediate evaluation.	
	▪ If the patient is suffering from constipation, the nurse should recommend a diet high in fiber and adequate fluid intake.[7]	
Labial adhesions	▪ The nurse should inquire about any associated symptoms occurring from the adhesions, such as vaginal discomfort, difficulty with urination, and/ or recurrent vaginal or urine infections.	▪ Topical steroid creams[5] ▪ Topical estrogen therapy[5]
	▪ The nurse should assess for adherence to medication regimens prescribed and if the patient has experienced any side effects.	
	▪ Treatment is typically continued until the adhesions resolve.	
	▪ Patients who have not noticed an improvement in adhesions and/or report side effects with medication should be seen in clinic for further evaluation.	

STIs, sexually transmitted infections.

➡ RED FLAGS

Pain: Patients with severe pain should be evaluated in the urgent care setting or an ED.

Concern for sexual abuse: Any suspicion of sexual abuse or trauma needs to be referred to the ED.

Vaginal trauma: If a vaginal trauma has occurred, such as a straddle injury, the patient should be evaluated in the ED, especially if the patient is experiencing heavy vaginal bleeding.

Retained foreign body: An urgent office visit should be offered for pediatric patients experiencing a malodorous, gree- tinged, and/or blood-tinged discharge. This may be concerning for a foreign body in the area, and prompt removal is necessary to prevent subsequent vaginal infections.

⊙ SPECIAL POPULATION CONSIDERATIONS

Patients with developmental delay: These patients may not be able to describe their pain or direct a caregiver to the area of concern. This population may also be at a higher risk for sexual abuse. These patients should always be evaluated by a provider if a caregiver voices concerns for vulvovaginitis.

TABLE 22.3 Commonly Prescribed Medications for Treatment of Pediatric Vulvovaginitis

Medicine	Common Side Effects*
Antibiotics	▪ Antibiotics should only be given for known pathogen from a culture. ▪ Contact the provider for side effect recommendations.
Barrier creams	▪ Barrier creams and ointments can be used with an identified condition. ▪ Ensure they are being administered the way the prescription was written and for the length of time ordered.
Estrogen creams	▪ Irritation, hyperpigmentation, bleeding, breast bud formation ▪ Side effects are uncommon. ▪ Proper application and limited duration of treatment can help decrease side effects.[5]
Steroid creams	▪ Thinning of skin
Stool softeners	▪ Stool softeners should be taken with adequate water intake to help the medications work.

*Consult with a provider regarding any patient-reported side effects.

SUMMARY

■ Vulvovaginitis can occur at any age with many reasons for symptoms.

■ In most instances, vulvovaginitis has a nonspecific cause.[8]

■ It is generally recommended to use a barrier ointment like petroleum jelly, good handwashing, and good vulvar hygiene, like wiping front to back.

RELATED PROTOCOL

■ Chapter 21: Urinary Concerns

References

1. Brander E, McQuillan S. Prepubertal vulvovaginitis. *CMAJ*. 2018;190(26):E800. doi:10.1503/cmaj.180004
2. Cemek F, Odabas D, Senel U, et al. Personal hygiene and vulvovaginitis in prepubertal children. *J Pediatr Adolesc Gynecol*. 2016;29:223–227. doi:10.1016/j.jpag.2015.07.002
3. Oquendo Del Toro HM, Hoefgen HR. Vulvovaginitis. In: Kliegman RM, et al. *Nelson Textbook of Pediatrics*. 21st ed. Elsevier Inc; 2020:2844–2851.
4. Stricker T. Vulvovaginitis. *Paediatr Child Health*. 2010;20(3):143–145. doi:10.1016/j.paed.2009.10.002
5. Bacon JL, Romano ME, Quint EH. Clinical recommendation: labial adhesions. *J Pediatr Adolesc Gynecol*. Oct, 2015;28(5):405–409. doi:10.1016/j.jpag.2015.04.010
6. Burkhart CN, Burkhart CG. Assessment of frequency, transmission, and genitourinary complications of enterobiasis (pinworms). *Int J Dermatol*. 2005;44(10): 837. doi:10.1111/j.1365-4632.2004.02332.x
7. Tabbers MM, DiLorenzo C, Berger MY, et al. Evaluation and treatment of functional constipation in infants and children: evidence-based recommendations from ESPGHAN and NASPGHAN. *J Pediatr Gastroenterol Nutr*. 2014;58(2):258. doi:10.1097/MPG.0000000000000266
8. Belna S, Gomez-Lobo V. Management of vulvar pain not associated with vulvovaginitis in prepubertal girls. *J Pediatr Adolesc Gynecol*. 2015;28(2):e68. doi:10.1016/j.jpag.2015.02.091

23

ADOLESCENT VULVOVAGINITIS AND VAGINAL DISCHARGE
Jennifer Kurkowski

INTRODUCTION

Vaginal discharge is characterized by fluid that comes out of the vagina. Normal vaginal discharge is due to endocervical secretions, vaginal flora, and epithelial cells sloughing.

Many women will have a small amount of vaginal discharge daily and can be 1 to 4 mL in volume per 24 hours. Normal discharge can increase 2 weeks prior to a normal menstrual cycle starting, or if a patient is using hormonal contraceptives the discharge may become thicker or even decrease over time. Normal discharge is typically clear to white and can be thick. This discharge is typically odorless.[1]

Many females will develop a vaginal infection during their lifetime. These symptoms can include vaginal discharge associated with change in color or volume, itching, odor, discomfort, burning, spotting, dysuria, and spotting.[2] Laboratory documentation should be used prior to treatment, as many vaginal symptoms can be nonspecific.[3] These laboratory tests include saline microscopy, cultures, DNA hybridization probes, gram stain, rapid antigen test, nucleic acid amplification tests, and microscopy with and without potassium hydroxide (KOH).

CLINICAL PEARL BOX

Common vaginal infections include both vulvovaginal candidiasis and bacterial vaginosis (BV).

Common sexually transmitted infections (STIs) include trichomoniasis, gonorrhea, and chlamydia.

COMMON PATIENT CONCERNS

- Vaginal discharge
- Vaginal itching
- Vulvar irritation
- Vaginal pain/discomfort

(O) KEY QUESTIONS TO ASK

Vaginal discharge

- When did the patient first notice the discharge?
- What is the quantity and color of your discharge?
- Is it associated with any itching, discomfort, burning?
- Is it associated with an odor? If so, can the patient describe the odor? Does the patient wear tampons, and if so, is there any chance of a retained tampon?
- Is it associated with dyspareunia or postcoital bleeding?
- Is the patient experiencing any vaginal bleeding, pelvic pain, or fever?
- Is the patient sexually active?

Vaginal Itching

- Is the patient experiencing any discharge changes? If so, can the patient describe the discharge (color, consistency, odor, etc.)?
- Is there any associated erythema or edema?
- Is the patient sexually active?
- Has the patient used any new soaps or products?
- Has the patient taken antibiotics recently?

Vaginal pain

- Is the patient experiencing any discharge changes? If so, can the patient describe the discharge (color, consistency, odor, etc.)?
- Is there any associated erythema or edema?
- Is the patient sexually active?
- Is it associated with intercourse or urination?
- What is the patient's pain on a numeric pain scale?
- Are there any visible lesions, ulcerations, or skin anomalies noted?

PATIENT ASSESSMENT

TABLE 23.1 Acute Symptoms of Adolescent Vulvovaginitis

Acute Symptoms	Intervention/Delegation	Commonly Prescribed Medicine
Malodorous vaginal discharge	▪ Malodorous vaginal discharge consistent with a fishy odor may be a sign of BV. It is often associated with a white/grey-toned discharge. Please schedule a clinic visit for evaluation.[4] ▪ Malodorous vaginal discharge may be a sign of an STI in patients who are sexually active. Please schedule a clinic visit for evaluation. ▪ Malodorous discharge can be a sign of a retained foreign body in the vagina. If there is any chance of a retained tampon or any type of foreign body, the patient must be seen in clinic for prompt evaluation and removal.	▪ Antibiotics
Discolored vaginal discharge	**Yellow-/green-tinged discharge** ▪ This can be a sign of vaginal trichomoniasis. Other symptoms may include an odor, pain with intercourse, dysuria, erythema, and/or postcoital bleeding. ▪ Please schedule a clinic evaluation for prompt evaluation/treatment. **Dark brown discharge** ▪ This can be related to intermenstrual bleeding or a sign of cervicitis caused by an STI. ▪ Assess whether the patient is using hormonal contraception, as it may be breakthrough spotting related to their contraceptive option. See appropriate chapter for further recommendations. ▪ Please schedule a clinic visit for evaluation.	▪ Antibiotics
Vaginal discharge with pelvic pain and/or a fever	▪ These can be signs of PID. Most cases are caused by gonorrhea and chlamydia. ▪ Other symptoms may include pain with intercourse, postcoital bleeding.	▪ Anti-fungal agents

(continued)

TABLE 23.1 Acute Symptoms of Adolescent Vulvovaginitis (*continued*)

Acute Symptoms	Intervention/Delegation	Commonly Prescribed Medicine
	▦ Please schedule an urgent clinic visit. If patient is acutely ill, please refer the patient to the ED for evaluation.	
Vulvar irritation	▦ Vulvar irritation associated with a vaginal discharge may be a sign of vulvovaginal candidiasis (vaginal yeast infection). As discussed above, laboratory findings and physical exam should be done prior to treatment so please schedule a clinic visit.[2] Other commonly associated symptoms include a thick, curd-like discharge, vaginal itching, and erythema. ▦ Vulvar itching may be hygiene related. The nurse should assess which type of soap the patient is washing with and frequency of bathing. It is typically recommended to wash once daily with an unscented soap. ▦ Vaginal irritation may also occur from friction during intercourse. The nurse may suggest trying lubrication during intercourse.	▦ Barrier creams ▦ Anti-fungal agents
Vaginal itching	▦ Vaginal itching associated with a vaginal discharge may be a sign of vulvovaginal candidiasis (yeast infection). As discussed above, laboratory findings and physical exam should be done prior to treatment so please schedule a clinic visit.[2] Other commonly associated symptoms include a thick, curd-like discharge, vaginal itching, and erythema. ▦ Vulvar itching may be hygiene related. The nurse should assess which type of soap the patient is washing with and frequency of bathing. ▦ It is typically recommended to wash once daily with an unscented soap.	▦ Anti-fungal agents ▦ Barrier creams ▦ Topical steroid creams

BV, bacterial vaginosis; PID, pelvic inflammatory disease; STI, sexually transmitted infection.

TABLE 23.2 Chronic Symptoms of Adolescent Vulvovaginitis

Chronic Symptoms	Intervention/Delegation	Commonly Prescribed Medicine
Daily vaginal discharge that is white to clear and odorless	▪ Provide reassurance that the patient may be experiencing normal, physiological discharge. ▪ If the patient is having any associated symptoms or has noticed a change in amount/consistency of discharge, assist the patient in making an appointment for further evaluation. ▪ If the patient is sexually active, offer an appointment for STI testing and encourage the patient to always use condoms.	None
Malodorous discharge	▪ If a patient has a persistent vaginal odor, **please schedule an appointment for further evaluation.** ▪ The nurse should assess for any new changes associated with the discharge, whether or not the patient is sexually active.	▪ Antibiotics
Vaginal itching	▪ The nurse should reinforce appropriate hygiene measures. The nurse should assess which contact irritants the patient has been avoiding and help identify any additional triggers. ▪ For patients with known or suspected lichen sclerosis, the nurse should inquire on which treatment the patient is using, duration of treatment, and any response to treatment. ▪ If the patient has persistent vaginal itching, please schedule an appointment for further evaluation.	▪ Anti-fungal agents ▪ Barrier creams ▪ Topical steroid creams
Vaginal pain	▪ If the patient is sexually active, inquire about lubrication use during intercourse. ▪ Please schedule an appointment for further evaluations	▪ NSAIDs ▪ Lubricant ▪ Stool softeners

NSAIDs, nonsteroidal anti-inflammatory drugs; STI, sexually transmitted infection.

➡ RED FLAGS

Pelvic inflammatory disease **(PID)**: Pelvic pain associated with discharge and/or a fever can be a sign of PID. Prompt recognition and treatment is vital, as PID can lead to infertility. Patients experiencing symptoms of this should be evaluated as soon as possible and may need to be referred to the ED.

TABLE 23.3 Commonly Prescribed Medicines for Treatment of Adolescent Vulvovaginitis

Medicine	Common Side Effects*
Over-the-counter intravaginal agents for candidiasis infections	Vulvovaginal burning, pruritus, soreness, swelling (local reactions)[5]
Oral fluconazole	Nausea, headaches, rash, vomiting, diarrhea, dizziness[6]
Intravaginal metronidazole	Local irritation, erythema, pruritus, burning, stinging[7]
Oral metronidazole	Nausea, vomiting, epigastric discomfort, diarrhea, metallic taste, rash, headache, dizziness, dark-colored urine[7]
Oral clindamycin	Rash, diarrhea, nausea, vomiting, abdominal pain, pruritus, metallic taste[8]
Ceftriaxone	Local injection site reaction, diarrhea[9]
Doxycycline	Headache, nausea, rash, diarrhea, vomiting, photosensitivity[10]
NSAIDs	Nausea, dyspepsia

NSAID, nonsteroidal anti-inflammatory drug.

*For side effects related to medications please notify the patient's provider. Some alternative therapies may be considered for treatment. If an anaphylactic-like reaction occurs, the patient should be referred to the ED immediately.

⊙ SPECIAL POPULATION CONSIDERATIONS

Immunocompromised patients: Patients who are immunocompromised, such as HIV positive or patients with diabetes, may be at greater risk for vaginal infections.

Patients with developmental delay: Patients with developmental delay may be at a higher risk for sexual abuse.

SUMMARY

■ Vaginal complaints are a common concern for many patients.

■ Reviewing normal symptoms versus signs of infections is important.

■ Most vaginal complaints need to be addressed during a clinic visit, but the nurse can assist patients in recommended comfort and hygiene measures while awaiting a visit appointment.

■ The nurse should be aware of signs of PID, as this needs to be treated urgently since it can lead to infertility.

RELATED PROTOCOLS

- Chapter 19: STD Exposure
- Chapter 13: Acute Pelvic Pain
- Chapter 14: Chronic Pelvic Pain

References

1. Anderson MR, Klink K, Cohrssen A. Evaluation of vaginal complaints. *JAMA*. 2004;291(11):1368. doi:10.1001/jama.291.11.1368
2. Workowski KA, Bolan GA. Sexually transmitted diseases treatment guidelines, 2015. Centers for Disease Control and Prevention. *MMWR Recomm Rep*. 2015; 64(RR-03):1.
3. Landers DV, Wiesenfeld HC, Heine RP, Krohn MA, Hillier SL. Predictive value of the clinical diagnosis of lower genital tract infection in women. *Am J Obstet Gynecol*. 2004;190(4):1004. doi:10.1016/j.ajog.2004.02.015
4. Fredricks DN, Fiedler TL, Marrazzo JM. Molecular identification of bacteria associated with bacterial vaginosis. *N Engl J Med*. 2005;353(18):1899. doi:10.1056/NEJMoa043802
5. Miconazole. *Lexi-Drugs*. *Lexicomp*. Riverwoods, IL: Wolters Kluwer Health, Inc. http://online.lexi.com. Accessed July 30, 2019.
6. Fluconazole. *Lexi-Drugs*. *Lexicomp*. Riverwoods, IL: Wolters Kluwer Health, Inc. http://online.lexi.com. Accessed July 30, 2019.
7. Metronidazole. *Lexi-Drugs*. *Lexicomp*. Riverwoods, IL: Wolters Kluwer Health, Inc. http://online.lexi.com. Accessed July 30, 2019.
8. Clindamycin. *Lexi-Drugs*. *Lexicomp*. Riverwoods, IL: Wolters Kluwer Health, Inc. http://online.lexi.com. Accessed July 30, 2019.
9. Ceftriaxone. *Lexi-Drugs*. *Lexicomp*. Riverwoods, IL: Wolters Kluwer Health, Inc. http://online.lexi.com. Accessed July 30, 2019.
10. Doxycycline. *Lexi-Drugs*. *Lexicomp*. Riverwoods, IL: Wolters Kluwer Health, Inc. http://online.lexi.com. Accessed July 30, 2019.

APPENDIX
Human Papillomavirus Vaccine

The human papillomavirus (HPV) vaccine currently protects against up to 90% of HPV related cancers, along with genital warts.[1] The Centers for Disease Control (CDC) currently recommends patients receive the vaccine at 11 to 12 years of age and complete two doses given 6 months apart.[2] The vaccine has recently been approved for use for patients up to 45 years of age, although the vaccine guidelines are still surrounding patients between ages 9 and 26.[2] Table A.1 shows the recommended schedule for the vaccine.

TABLE A.1 HPV Vaccine Schedule

Age Range	Number of Doses Needed	Recommended Dosing Interval	Minimum Interval Between Doses	Maximum Interval Between Doses
9–14 years of age	2	0, 6–12-month schedule.	The minimum interval is 5 months between doses.	There is no maximum interval between doses, so if a series is interrupted, it does not need to be restarted.
15–26 years of age (and some adults up to 45 years of age)	3	0, 1–2 month, 6–12-month schedule.	The minimum interval is 4 weeks between the first and second dose, 12 weeks between the second and third dose, and 5 months between first and third dose.	There is no maximum interval between doses, so if a series is interrupted, it does not need to be restarted.

HPV, human papillomavirus.

Source: Centers for Disease Control and Prevention. HPV vaccine schedule and dosing. https://www.cdc.gov/hpv/hcp/schedules-recommendations.html. Accessed May 5, 2020.

TABLE A.2 Recommended Schedule for HPV in Immunocompromised Patients

Medical Condition	Series to Follow
HIV	All patients with HIV should receive three doses to ensure adequate benefit of the vaccine.
Cancer	Patients immunocompromised from cancer should receive three doses of the HPV vaccine to ensure adequate benefit of the vaccine.
Autoimmune disease	Patients immunocompromised from certain autoimmune diseases should receive three doses of the HPV vaccine to ensure adequate benefit of the vaccine.
Posttransplantation	Patients immunocompromised following organ transplants should receive three doses of the HPV vaccine to ensure adequate benefit of the vaccine.
Immunosuppressive medications	Patients immunocompromised from certain medications should receive three doses of the HPV vaccine to ensure adequate benefit of the vaccine.
Diabetes	Patients with diabetes can follow the usual guidelines for age. Special dosing is not needed.

HPV, human papillomavirus.

Source: Centers for Disease Control and Prevention. HPV vaccine schedule and dosing. https://www.cdc.gov/hpv/hcp/schedules-recommendations.html. Accessed May 5, 2020.

HPV VACCINE SCHEDULE IN SPECIAL POPULATIONS AGES 9 TO 26

The CDC recommends following the three-dose interval for immunocompromised patients to help ensure adequate benefit is received from the vaccine (Table A.2). The nurse should check with the provider regarding the schedule for patients with chronic medical conditions.[2]

COMMON SIDE EFFECTS

- Local pain, redness, and swelling at injection site.[3]
- Feelings of light-headedness or dizziness following administration of injection.
- Syncope (most common in those who faint with any vaccine).

Safety concerns: There is robust data supporting the safety of the HPV vaccine. Regardless, patients may have questions regarding a link between the vaccine and specific medical conditions.

Autoimmune disease: Evidence does not support an association between autoimmune diseases and the HPV vaccine.[4–14]

Death: Evidence does not show the vaccine can cause death.[3]

Fertility: The CDC has not found any evidence between the vaccine and fertility or primary ovarian insufficiency.[14]

Chronic fatigue syndrome (CFS): Studies have not supported risk of CFS in adolescent females who received the vaccine.[1,15–16]

References

1. Centers for Disease Control and Prevention. HPV cancers are preventable. https://www.cdc.gov/hpv/hcp/protecting-patients.html. Accessed May 5, 2020.
2. Centers for Disease Control and Prevention. HPV vaccine schedule and dosing. https://www.cdc.gov/hpv/hcp/schedules-recommendations.html. Accessed May 5, 2020.
3. Centers for Disease Control and Prevention. Vaccine safety. https://www.cdc.gov/vaccinesafety/index.html?CDC_AA_refVal=https%3A%2F%2Fwww.cdc.gov%2Fvaccinesafety%2Findex.htm. Accessed May 5, 2020.
4. Andrews N, Stowe J, Miller E. No increased risk of Guillain-Barre syndrome after human papilloma virus vaccine: a self-controlled case-series study in England. *Vaccine*. 2017;35(13):1729–1732. doi:10.1016/j.vaccine.2017.01.076
5. Arnheim-Dahlstrom L, Pasternak B, Svanstrom H, Sparen P, Hviid A. Autoimmune, neurological, and venous thromboembolic adverse events after immunisation of adolescent girls with quadrivalent human papillomavirus vaccine in Denmark and Sweden: cohort study. *BMJ*. 2013;347:f5906. doi:10.1136/bmj.f5906
6. Chao C, Klein NP, Velicer CM, et al. Surveillance of autoimmune conditions following routine use of quadrivalent human papillomavirus vaccine. *J Intern Med*. 2012;271(2):193–203. doi:10.1111/j.1365-2796.2011.02467.x
7. Deceuninck G, Sauvageau C, Gilca V, Boulianne N, De Serres G. Absence of association between Guillain-Barre syndrome hospitalizations and HPV-vaccine. *Expert Rev Vaccines*. 2018;17(1):99–102. doi:10.1080/14760584.2018.1388168
8. Gee J, Sukumaran L, Weintraub E. Risk of Guillain-Barre Syndrome following quadrivalent human papillomavirus vaccine in the Vaccine Safety Datalink. *Vaccine*. 2017;35(43):5756–5758. doi:10.1016/j.vaccine.2017.09.009
9. Grimaldi-Bensouda L, Guillemot D, Godeau B, et al. Autoimmune disorders and quadrivalent human papillomavirus vaccination of young female subjects. *J Intern Med*. 2014;275(4):398–408. doi:10.1111/joim.12155
10. Grimaldi-Bensouda L, Rossignol M, Kone-Paut I, et al. Risk of autoimmune diseases and human papilloma virus (HPV) vaccines: six years of case-referent surveillance. *J Autoimmun*. 2017;79:84–90. doi:10.1016/j.jaut.2017.01.005
11. Hviid A, Svanstrom H, Scheller NM, Gronlund O, Pasternak B, Arnheim-Dahlstrom L. Human papillomavirus vaccination of adult women and risk of autoimmune and neurological diseases. *J Intern Med*. 2018;283(2):154–165. doi:10.1111/joim.12694
12. Klein NP, Goddard K, Lewis E, et al. Long term risk of developing type 1 diabetes after HPV vaccination in males and females. *Vaccine*. 2019;37(14):1938–1944. doi:10.1016/j.vaccine.2019.02.051
13. Liu EY, Smith LM, Ellis AK, et al. Quadrivalent human papillomavirus vaccination in girls and the risk of autoimmune disorders: the Ontario Grade 8 HPV Vaccine Cohort Study. *CMAJ*. 2018;190(21):E648–e55. doi:10.1503/cmaj.170871
14. Naleway AL, Mittendorf KF, Irving SA, et al. Primary ovarian insufficiency and adolescent vaccination. *Pediatrics*. 2018;142(3):e20180943. doi:10.1542/peds.2018-0943

15. Feiring B, Laake I, Bakken IJ, et al. HPV vaccination and risk of chronic fatigue syndrome/myalgic encephalomyelitis: A nationwide register-based study from Norway. *Vaccine.* 2017;35(33):4203–4212. doi:10.1016/j.vaccine.2017.06.031

16. Centers for Disease Control and Prevention. Vaccine adverse event reporting system (VAERS). https://www.cdc.gov/vaccinesafety/ensuringsafety/monitoring/vaers/index.html. Accessed May 5, 2020.

INDEX

Printed in the United States
by Baker & Taylor Publisher Services